FOLKS

FOLKS

Memoirs of a Public Health Nurse

BY LINDA CURD LAKER, RN, BSN

WITH KATHY GROGAN, BA, EdM

Printed in the United States of America

Designed by Megan Katsanevakis

Library of Congress Control Number: 2020923475

ISBN: 978-1-951568-89-4 (Hardcover edition)

ISBN: 978-1-951568-11-5 (Softcover edition)

PHOTO CREDITS: Page 6 courtesy, *The Evening Tribune*;

page 60 courtesy, *The Evening Tribune*.

All other photos courtesy Linda Curd Laker.

SMALL
BATCH
BOOKS

493 SOUTH PLEASANT STREET

AMHERST, MASSACHUSETTS 01002

413.230.3943

SMALLBATCHBOOKS.COM

To my dear husband, Jim, who is my best friend
and means everything to me.

Author's note:

This is a work of creative nonfiction. I have tried to recreate events, locales, and conversations to the best of my recollection. When necessary, I have filled in gaps, while keeping in mind the essence of what actually happened. While the stories in this book are true, names have been omitted and identifying details have been changed to protect the privacy of the people involved.

CONTENTS

My First Day: November 1977 - xi

Chapter 1 - Why I Became a Public Health Nurse - 1

Chapter 2 - Travel Woes - 7

Chapter 3 - Animal Tales - 17

Chapter 4 - Different Strokes - 33

Chapter 5 - Dangers - 45

Chapter 6 - Caregivers - 49

Chapter 7 - Sick Children - 59

Chapter 8 - Death - 65

Chapter 9 - Homes Reflect Their Owners - 73

Chapter 10 - Changes in Public Health Nursing Over the Years - 83

Chapter 11 - Special Cases - 89

Chapter 12 - Lessons Learned: Final Thoughts on My Career - 107

My Last Day: September 2013 - 109

Acknowledgments - 111

MY FIRST DAY:

November 1977

AFTER BRUSHING THE snow off my little green and white Chevy Monza, I put my bag, hand-drawn maps of the area, and travel directions to each of my destinations in the car. As I settle myself behind the wheel, decked out in my navy and white uniform, including a hat, I feel so many emotions: fear, anxiety, excitement, and eagerness. I study the map and directions to my first destination, start the car, and begin a journey that takes thirty-six years to complete.

As I navigate the streets and head into rural Western New York, I wonder what I will find when I reach that first home. I have been well-trained and feel prepared. That morning I packed my bag, hopefully with everything I would need for the day's visits: my newspapers, my aprons, gloves, syringes, blood pressure cuff, and stethoscope—even slippers, suggested to me by my mentor, to put on as a courtesy once I remove my boots so that I don't track dirt through a person's home.

Despite my training and preparation, I still feel a bit nervous walking up to that first door. I remind myself that I am not selling anything or intruding into these people's lives. I am there to help them. So I knock. When the door opens, the homeowner sees my uniform and bag and smiles, welcoming me, glad that a public health nurse is there to provide the care necessary to help a family member get better.

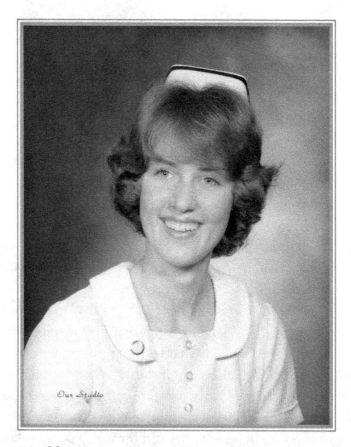

My nursing graduation picture, May 1975.

ONE

WHY I BECAME A PUBLIC HEALTH NURSE

If possible, find a way to do what you love to do.

IN SEPTEMBER 1960, a little six-year-old girl found herself in the hospital. She had been at a best friend's birthday party the week before, but when she returned home she didn't feel well. She was suffering from a fever, lethargy, and abdominal cramps. When the usual home remedies failed, she was admitted to the hospital, where she was diagnosed with a virus that had settled in her colon and created a bowel obstruction, known as volvulus. This condition required a bowel resection and a lengthy hospital stay of a month. Being in a ward with other children was frightening. She was in a strange place surrounded by sick children—including one who couldn't see, as her eyes were bandaged the whole time she was there—and the hustle and bustle of the hospital. As you may have guessed, this little girl was me.

Compared to many of the children, I was fortunate in that my family came to visit me daily. Mom came every morning and stayed through lunch, then Grandma would show up. At dinnertime, Dad would arrive, followed by Grandpa after dinner.

One night Grandpa brought all the children on the ward metal pinwheels. When we pressed the lever on the bottom, the wheel would go round and round and make sparks in our dark room, entertaining us and the nurses too. When it was time to leave, Grandpa would walk me down to the TV room, where all the other kids were, and he'd say, "Now, don't cry. Be a big girl. Your mommy will be back in the morning." Then he'd put on his fedora (which now hangs in my kitchen) and depart. I was brave—because Grandpa told me to be.

In between and during my family visits, I found myself intently watching the nurses as they performed their duties, comforted me and the other children, and let us know everything would be all right. These women—and they all were women—made a lasting impression on me at a time when I needed reassurance. They were so gentle and kind. I thought, "This is what I want to do: Make a sweet little girl, alone in a strange place and fearful of everything, feel safe, loved, and cared for." And in time, I did.

I was not a gifted student. In elementary school, the comments on my report card were always, "Linda is a delightful young lady who could do much better if she applied herself." I hated sitting still for six hours a day and found reading and spelling challenging. In seventh grade, when I started changing classes every forty-five minutes, my grades began to improve. However, I was worried about succeeding with the more rigorous middle school coursework. I went to my guidance counselor with concerns about reading, and he enrolled me in a speed-reading program. That program helped, but I still struggled. It wasn't until later in life that I realized I'm dyslexic.

In high school, the addition of sports, science, labs, and new friends brightened my outlook on school even more. I excelled at practical applications and hands-on experiences. Most of all, I liked organization and problem-solving. Concerned that I might not scholastically be up to the challenge of further education, I was tentative in my pursuit of nursing and attended the local two-year college to acquire an associate of applied science degree. Luckily, within two months, I was already working with patients.

In my second year of college, I took an EMT course with all the local firemen and ambulance crews. This course was a real eye-opener for me. Though I had more knowledge about disease processes and injuries, they all knew the protocols and equipment of an ambulance. This was before the implementation of 9-1-1, and there were at least forty different phone numbers that corresponded with the different towns where our patients lived. Each public health nurse traveled with a list of all the numbers of emergency services connected to the various townships. My EMT training helped me to navigate the various local systems and facilitate transportation of a patient to the hospital. I knew the procedures for getting a patient on the gurney safely, as well as what details would be needed by the ambulance crew. In my nursing practice, when a patient had to be transported, I knew to have the patient's most recent vitals and list of medications already written out, and to move the furniture in the home for easy access.

The practical aspect of the associate-degree curriculum, combined with my EMT coursework, reinforced the college bookwork, which, in turn, resulted in good grades. My educational progress sparked a desire to extend my knowledge, and I applied to another school to pursue my bachelor of science in nursing. It was during this time that I was immersed in a semester of public health nursing. This experience spoke deeply to my desire to really connect with people in a meaningful way. Out in the community, driving from house to house, caring for folks in their own environment—fabulous! This was what I was meant to do. This was my path.

Being a public health nurse would require more experience and knowledge than I could gain in college. Out in the field, a public health nurse is on her own. There is no staff to ask for help. It's just you, the family, occasionally a home health aide, and the doctor on the phone. To get the additional tools I would need, I worked nights at a local hospital while pursuing my degree. I learned so much during these late-night hours, witnessing birth and death and honing my medical skills.

Working nights in a small-town hospital is an experience. Night shifts, which are vastly different from day shifts, are composed of just a skeleton crew. The nurse on the floor provides not only the standard nursing required—oral medications, IV therapy, dosage changes, and catheter care—but also respiratory therapy treatments, blood draws as needed, and comfort care.

Folks are born and die in the wee hours of the night. Before I set out to treat patients in their homes, I needed to experience these momentous life events in the safe environment of a hospital. I asked my supervisor if I could observe any births that occurred during the quiet hours of the night shift, and she readily agreed. Each time I observed this magical beginning of life, I was moved to tears. There is nothing more awe-inspiring than the entry cry of a new human being.

Death is entirely different. The first time I put a stethoscope on the chest of someone who had passed, I was startled at the absence of sound. The silence was absolute and opened a different door in me. Being with a living soul one moment and feeling that soul pass—words cannot express the experience. It's astounding. The lifeless body immediately feels different. I would bathe the patient, take out all the tubes, and make the person presentable for the family to see before sending what was now just a body to the morgue.

With my hospital experience and my bachelor's degree in hand, I was ready to embark on my career. In 1977, I started in public health as a county nurse. I loved it from day one—there was never a dull moment.

I not only learned so much about treating the illnesses of my patients, but in many cases, I also became almost a part of the family.

As I look back on my thirty-six years in the job, I reflect on the many lessons I learned and, most of all, on the folks who invited me into their homes and inspired me with their courage in the face of adversity. I hope by sharing their stories, I can pass along some of the joy and inspiration they brought me throughout my career.

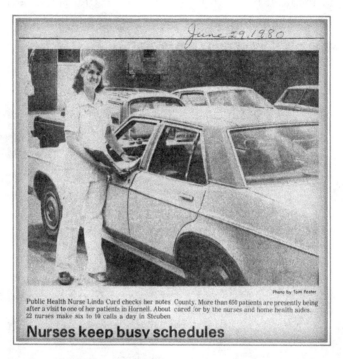

June 29, 1980

Photo by Tom Foster

Public Health Nurse Linda Curd checks her notes after a visit to one of her patients in Hornell. About 22 nurses make six to 10 calls a day in Steuben County. More than 650 patients are presently being cared for by the nurses and home health aides.

Nurses keep busy schedules

ME IN UNIFORM AT MY CAR, JUNE 29, 1980.
I DID NOT HAVE MY HAT ON (IT WAS IN THE CAR),
AND I WAS REPRIMANDED BY MY SUPERVISOR.

TWO
TRAVEL WOES

Be Prepared.

OVER MANY YEARS of public health nursing, I learned the importance of being prepared. Since the job requires traveling in all kinds of weather to all kinds of places, being ready for anything is especially important. Yes, my various experiences in college and the hospital did much to prepare me for the work, but nothing beats actual on-the-job experience.

The universal uniform for a public health nurse was navy and white. When I first started working for the county, we were given a uniform allowance and had to purchase our uniforms from the official public health nursing Hopkins catalogue, which still exists today. I mostly chose to wear skirts, jackets, blouses, and jumpers with navy tights. It seemed more comfortable and suitable for bending, stooping, and maneuvering around patients. Each day, I would go home, immediately change, and put the uniform in the wash. I never wanted to inadvertently bring anything into my home from the "workplace," especially pests like fleas, scabies, and mites—all obviously unwanted.

My first nursing director was very strict, insisting that we also wear the official navy blue hat, which we did, except in the winter, when we were allowed to wear something warmer. We all wore the same navy blue coat with a zip-in lining for colder weather, but it was really more like a raincoat and not that warm. It was truly inadequate for the blustery, snowy winters, so I started dressing in layers: undershirt, blouse, jumper, cardigan, and coat. I could peel off my coat and sweater once I entered the patient's home.

One day, I was working on discharge planning at the hospital, which involves meeting with nurses and seeing prospective patients before they are sent home. I was on my way to the medical-surgical floors to meet with patients when the elevator opened, and a man got on. He took in my appearance—I had on the full uniform regalia, complete with pins, name tag on my lapel, and the navy hat—and promptly asked what airline I worked for. Mind you, this small hospital was seventy miles from the closest airport, but I could see his point.

Later, when a new director took over, the impractical regulation nursing hats and coats were no longer mandatory. We were allowed to choose our own coats as long as they were black or blue. I swapped out the nurse's cap for a warmer navy knit hat.

The most important part of the nursing uniform was the "nursing bag." It was black leather, similar to a doctor's bag, with a flap closure on the top. We would check our bags and pack them for the day, knowing how many and what type of visits we would be making. In the early years, the majority of our visits were assessment visits, injections, dressings, and maybe a blood draw. Then I would fold newspapers in a certain way to fit under the bag flap, one for each visit.

The most important rule regarding our bags was: *Never place your bag on the floor in any home, and always have a barrier between your bag and your environment to prevent the transmission of germs and critters from home to home.* This is what the papers were for. As time went on, my barrier evolved. I switched out the newspapers for a roll of cheap white garbage bags. Finally, I settled on Hopkins large waterproof blue pads that were superior to the other methods. The agency found them too expensive and wouldn't pay for them, so I bought them myself—a hundred at a time—and used them right up to retirement. When a different nurse would make a home visit to my patients, especially children, they would ask, "Where's your blue pad?" It made me realize what patients noticed, but I never did explain to them the pad's purpose.

As the patients became more acute and the procedures more complicated, our bags became larger. I needed to carry more than a blood pressure cuff and stethoscope. Supplies were usually sent directly to patients' homes, and I would carry the essentials to complete the job, such as sterile gloves, Q-tips, syringes, different needle options, a blood-draw kit, nail clippers, Kelly clamp (similar to needle-nose pliers), and extra IV tubing. I also had a container in my car with dressings in every size, catheters, Kling (gauze), irrigation sets, and the like. The worst thing in the world was to have a situation arise at a patient's home and not be prepared for it. It took a few years to figure out exactly what I needed to have with me at all times, but after I did, I was prepared for almost any eventuality.

I started with the agency in November of 1977, and what a winter to start public health nursing! Being the new kid, I was assigned to cover Christmas Day. Holidays were usually quiet, since most folks had family visiting and didn't want a home visit unless it was something they couldn't manage. An injection, catheter change, or a complicated dressing were the main reasons for visits in those days. In the seventies and eighties, we didn't do home IV therapy or many of the complicated dressings that are done now.

I did have an assignment on that first Christmas morning. We had a blind patient whom we visited every morning to administer insulin (I believe we took care of her for over twenty years). Knowing I had this call to make, I decided to spend Christmas Eve with my mom, get up early, make the home visit, and then celebrate Christmas with my family.

Before Mom and I went out to spend Christmas Eve with friends, it started snowing. It was beautiful, like a glittery Christmas card, but not great for driving. So we each donned one of my mom's fur coats and walked three blocks to our friend's house for our Christmas Eve revelries. Our little town never looked so appropriately festive, with all the lights and soft snow falling and coating the trees and ground. I'll never forget it, or the day that followed.

On Christmas morning, Mom was up first and called to me, "Wow, there's a lot of snow. I don't think you're going anywhere." Well, that was not an option. I had to get to my patient by 9:30 a.m., and it was now 7:00 a.m. The main roads had been plowed, but our driveway and my car were buried at least three feet deep in snow. I dressed and started making telephone calls. First, I called my supervisor, who suggested that I call the sheriff's office. That office was no help, telling me to "Stay put." After trying a few other agencies to ask for some kind of assistance, I finally called our local fire department. They came to the rescue, hooking a chain to my Ford Granada (no four-wheel drive in this baby), and hauled it—still covered in snow—into the street, ready to be driven the seven miles to my patient. Just before I started down the street, my neighbor's son, who obviously had noticed all the commotion out front, came to the door and yelled, "Do you want company?" I eagerly responded "Yes," thankful to have someone with me on what could prove to be a hazardous journey. He came clomping out of his house in a pair of bright red, hard plastic ski boots with three clips, one for the ankle and two on the foot. Since he was visiting from Arizona, this was the only winter gear he had. I was a bit hesitant when he offered to drive, wondering how he could do it in those stiff boots, but he was able to manage it well.

With him behind the wheel, we started down the street with five-foot walls of snow on each side of the car. There was no traffic except emergency vehicles, and the only roads that were plowed were the main thoroughfares. All side streets were blocked or still being cleared at that time in the morning. The snow was so clean and white. I was astonished by how quiet it was! He got me safely to the city where my patient lived, but there was another obstacle.

Since only the main roads had been plowed—no parking lots, side-walks, or side roads—my patient's street was inaccessible. My neighbor's son got me as close to my patient's home as possible, and I waded the rest of the way through deep snow, powder flying with each step. I reflected that if I were five feet two I wouldn't have made it. As I was trudging up to her door, somewhat the worse for wear, a New York State Electric and Gas truck went by with one of my friends driving. He saw me, rolled down his window while grinning, wildly waved, and yelled, "Merry Christmas!" I knew this was his first Christmas as a dad, and he, like me, had to work. His warm greeting really made me smile, and I yelled back, "Merry Christmas to you, too!" That moment left a lasting impression on me, because there we were—just a few of us—conquering the elements and doing our jobs in the quiet and purity of the snow.

My patient lived in an upstairs apartment above a downtown store. I climbed the three flights of stairs to her door, knocked, and went into the kitchen without removing my coat. The apartment was dull and gray with not a Christmas decoration in sight. My patient was just as drab in her pale, flowered night dress covered with a threadbare cotton duster. Without a hello or a holiday greeting, she snapped, "Hurry up so I can eat my breakfast." I tried not to be offended by her tone, recognizing that she was most likely anxious due to the combination of holiday and blizzard, as well as fearful that I wasn't going to get to her. I went over to the sink, washed my hands, drew up the insulin, and gave her the injection. Then I wished her a Merry Christmas and headed out.

I lumbered back through my original footsteps toward the main road. My neighbor, who had been driving around because he couldn't park in the plowed part of the road, was right on time. He stopped long enough for me to get into the car, and we headed home. I was so fortunate to have him with me. There would have been nowhere for me to park, and the camaraderie of overcoming the treacherous conditions together made the day much more pleasant. My patient had no idea the effort it took to get to her, but I was thankful that I was able to do my job despite the many obstacles.

What an initiation into a career in public health! That winter, we had so much snow that the roads were closed twice. Those were the only times in my thirty-six-year career that we had snow days. We worked through all kinds of bad weather conditions, even during the ice storm of March 1991, described in a *New York Times* article by Robert McFadden as "The worst ice storm in decades." During the night, the temperature dropped, suddenly turning what had been rain into ice. The weight of ice on tree branches was so heavy that branches snapped, sounding like repeated gunshots. The next day, a fairyland of ice-coated trees surrounded us. As beautiful as it looked, it was extremely treacherous. Schools throughout the county and beyond were closed, but we weren't. Since I lived in town, I decided it was best to walk, very carefully, to the office instead of driving.

Though Western New York winters can be treacherous, our patients were usually considerate and worried about our safety. When the weather was bad, most of them would call the office to let us know if the roads in their areas had been plowed or not. We appreciated that. The folks who lived in the country were especially thoughtful, oftentimes saying, "I'll be all right today. Why don't you wait until tomorrow to visit?"

There was another time that bad conditions caused me problems.

I was in the country, making a home visit midmorning. I was feeling confident on the snowy back roads, as I had recently purchased a Chevy Blazer, my first four-wheel-drive vehicle. I was overly confident in what it could do. The patient's driveway had not been plowed, but I pulled right in anyway. While I was able to get into the driveway, there was no way I was getting out. The two and a half feet of snow under my vehicle did not allow any traction with my four-wheel drive. After trying unsuccessfully for twenty minutes to dislodge my Blazer, I finally sheepishly called my husband, who sold tow trucks for a living. He borrowed a tow truck from the dealership where he worked and came to pull me out.

Really, though, when I think about the abundance of iffy weather over my thirty-six years in the field, it's pretty amazing that I only got stuck that one time. He was my hero that day and continues to be.

After the early years, I was fortunate to have new, reliable vehicles for my journeys, but even a new vehicle can develop unexpected problems. I was once driving to visit my last patient of the day when—*bang!*—a flat on my right back tire. This happened in the country on River Road, which is desolate with no cell service. This was before services like OnStar. Only a few dwellings were scattered here and there, but none immediately nearby. My patient's home was about three miles farther up the road. I attempted to walk to where I could find help, and I did find a cabin, but no one was there. As I walked up the dirt driveway, I realized it was a seasonal camp: No lights were on and not a vehicle in sight. I decided the best option was to drive to my patient's home on my flat tire. I tried to minimize damage to the rim by inching the right wheels of my vehicle onto the softer shoulder. When I eventually arrived, I was able to call AAA from his landline, take care of him, and after the tire repair, drive home.

The next day I met a home health aide at a lovely gentleman's home, a long-term patient of the agency who was a quadriplegic. As I was caring for him, I told him my flat-tire story. I said, "What else was I going to do? It was a remote area. There was no cell reception. I had to drive on the flat." His response was priceless: "You coulda walked." I felt like he had slapped me in the face. The reality of his statement hit me that hard. After a few seconds of dead silence, all three of us started laughing. The choice to walk hadn't occurred to me. It really hadn't! This man, unable to use his legs, reminded me of how blessed I am and how minor my tire problem was!

While I mainly drove the Chevy Blazer for work because of the four-wheel drive and the back gate, making nursing supplies easy to access, an opportunity arose to purchase a vehicle that was a bit more "fun." My husband and I purchased a 1988 Cadillac Coupe de Ville, fully loaded, from a family member. To save miles on the Blazer, I decided to drive the Caddy during the summer months until October. The Caddy was powder blue with a white vinyl roof with gold trim and spoke wheels. This car was a real looker and attracted quite a bit of attention. A good friend of mine, who was a retired state trooper, met me in the

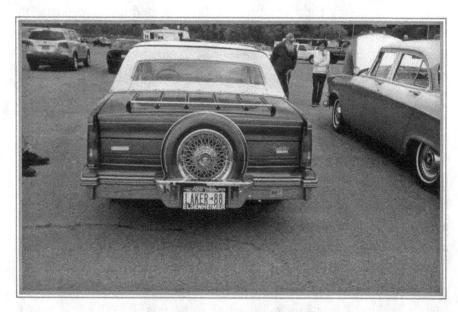

My 1988 Cadillac. What a car!

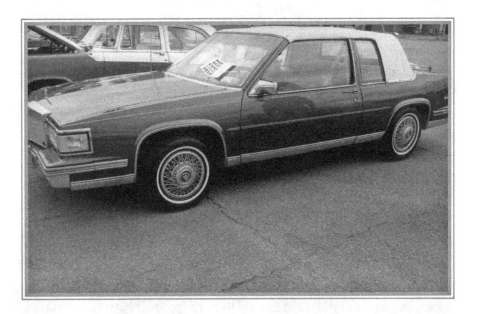

store one day and said, "Are you that beautiful woman in that blue and white car?" I loved answering, "Yes." That car was especially popular with my elderly gentlemen patients, and if I was visiting a patient in town, it was common for another patient to see that distinctive car and call out to invite me to stop by.

One day I was driving the Caddy in the country at about 2:00 p.m. when, all of a sudden, I felt a vibration coming from my front tire. I slowed down, and suddenly my right front tire totally blew up. The rubber shot up, hit the windshield, and the car pulled hard to the right, shaking to an abrupt stop. For a moment my hands just gripped the wheel. I was paralyzed. Eventually, I pulled myself together enough to get out of my car. While I was walking down the road trying to get cell reception, a very nice gentleman stopped to help. As he was changing my tire, I asked him why he happened to be there, and he explained that he lived up the road. To make conversation, I asked what he did for a living, and he explained that he didn't work, as he was on disability. Alarm bells started ringing in my head. I worried that he might have a bad back or weak heart. I exclaimed, "Please don't hurt yourself!" He looked me straight in the eye and told me, "No, my problem is mental." "Uh . . ." was all I managed to say. I thought to myself, Great. I'm in the middle of nowhere, with a disabled car, at the mercy of a gentleman with some unknown mental disability. The slight trepidation I felt, however, was unwarranted. This kind gentleman finished changing the tire and I was able to finish my day without further incident. I blame that moment of anxiety on too much *Forensic Files*, *20/20*, and *Law and Order* on TV.

When I think about all my years on the road, visiting patients in all kinds of weather, I feel fortunate that I only had a few problems, which were fairly easily resolved. My practical self told me to keep bottled water, granola bars, a small pillow, an army blanket, and calf-high boots in my car. Though I did what I could to be prepared, I have to be honest, I was lucky! I was blessed with a loving husband, reliable vehicles, and the kindness of strangers.

THREE

ANIMAL TALES

Learn to adapt to the patient's environment.
Beware of the animals!

WHEN MAKING HOME visits, you have to realize that pets are part of the environment, part of the family. Working in rural Western New York, I encountered both the usual and some unusual pets, each one with its own set of challenges.

Dogs and cats are perhaps the most common pets I encountered. I quickly discovered the importance of making the family dog your friend. I imagine every mailman, FedEx employee, and UPS driver would agree. Dogs own their homes. You are a guest or trespasser on their turf. They are protective not only of their property, but also of the patient you've come to tend. If a patient has had a recent extensive stay in the hospital, the dog is even more on guard against intruders, now that his beloved owner has returned. Fortunately, I love dogs. I believe they sense that in me, and for the most part, we get along. There are some breeds, however, that I would never turn my back on. Rottweilers and pit bulls are extremely strong and protective; oftentimes, I would have owners restrain them before my arrival.

Pets of all stripes—birds, cats, dogs, horses, or even tattooed bears, as you'll soon learn about—are all special to their owners. As a public health nurse and a guest in my patients' homes, I had the privilege of observing these connections many times over. Since my retirement, I miss the folks, but I also miss their dear furry—or feathery—friends.

In all my years of making home visits, I was bit only once. The dog was a female Dalmatian named Lady. Although Lady always barked a lot when I visited, she was never aggressive. On this particular day, I was seeing a teenage patient for a routine blood draw. The patient's parents were not at home, but I'm not sure that was a factor in what happened. After obtaining the sample, I packed up with Lady nowhere in sight. As I was leaving, Lady shot out of the bedroom and bit me on the side of my thigh, cutting right through my slacks. I was startled. I was dismayed. I was injured. Needless to say, it hurt!

But I had to deliver the blood sample to the hospital. So I quickly left, went to the hospital, dropped off the specimen, and then went to the restroom to assess my leg. I had a nice bruise already about the size of an orange with four distinct puncture wounds. I cleansed my leg well, called my supervisor to report the incident, and continued with my day. I think, in retrospect, that continuing to move about helped work out the soreness. Having to get the specimen to the hospital helped keep me calm.

When I contacted the family to follow up on the incident, I was reassured to learn that the dog was up to date on her rabies vaccinations. The family apologized profusely, musing on the fact that lately the dog had been atypically aggressive. Later that week, they informed me that Lady had died of an apparent brain tumor, which had most likely affected her vision. When I walked by the door, my shadow may have scared her, causing her to bite me in self-defense. Once I knew the rest of her story, I really couldn't blame her.

Most dogs are comical in their ways. I had a patient with a sweet, but deaf, Shar-Pei named Barney. He'd lost his hearing when the vet trimmed his ears and caused some nerve damage. I just had to make sure I was in his line of sight when I visited his owner. As long as Barney knew I was there, he was fine.

The patient had to have her nephrostomy tubes irrigated weekly. Since the tubes enter the kidney from the lower back, I would have to kneel down low to perform the irrigation. One day, while I was performing the irrigation, Barney came up behind me, placed his head on my shoulder, and just watched the entire time. So sweet.

Another time I was getting ready to leave and my beeper went off. To my—and the patient's—surprise, Barney reacted. Apparently the beeper's frequency pierced his deafness. Barney had such a look of ultimate amazement on his face at the recognition of sound in his silent world.

I followed this patient for quite a long time, and we became good friends. That Christmas, she gave me a magnum of champagne. What a gift! It came from one of the vineyards where her husband worked as an entomologist—one of the United States wineries that was grandfathered for the use of the word "champagne" for its bubbly.

Blackie was a chunky, black, extremely nervous dog that I would describe as a barking footstool with legs. His "parents" were elderly. "Dad" had had a stroke, and "Mom" was a sweet, little rotund lady who loved to bake. Whenever I visited them, Blackie would have a fit. I always gave him a biscuit to put an end to the barking. (I think all visitors gave him a biscuit when entering, which probably was the reason he was so heavy.) One day I made a routine visit to check on my patient, but there was no bark at the door, no "footstool" fit of greeting. Worried that something had happened to my fat friend, I inquired as to his whereabouts. The previous day, his owner had bought Blackie a knucklebone, and he got so excited, he had swallowed it whole. Surprisingly, he didn't choke; however, the bone was too big to pass, and Blackie had to have surgery. He did very well and was back to his old self in no time. Oftentimes, as I sat in the window seat to check my patient's vitals, Blackie would climb up, sit right next to me, lean against me, and be snoring away by the time I was ready to leave. He was my pal!

Sometimes being a nurse leads to some unusual patients—including the four-legged kind. Jethro was a big, lovable dog whose master was a severe diabetic. Having broken his leg, this young man was wheelchair bound. At the time of my visit, Jethro was tied up in front of the trailer. I was checking the patient's blood sugar, cast care, and circulation when we heard a terrible noise. It had to be the dog. I raced outside to discover that a car had passed too close to the trailer and somehow snagged Jethro's chain. The car had then dragged the dog about two or three feet before the chain came loose and the car drove on. It's possible that the driver wasn't aware of what had happened.

I unhooked the dog. Jethro was bleeding from the nose, mouth, and front paw. I brought him inside; I was surprised at how trusting he was. The poor thing was shook up, and his master was incapacitated, so I went to work. I cleaned up his face and mouth, then took a look at the paw and saw that a nail had been pulled out. I cleansed the paw with saline, then applied Betadine, covered it with a four-by-four gauze pad and wrapped it with Kling. That big, sweet dog never growled or flinched—he let me fix him up. On that particular visit, I think I did more for the dog than for the patient.

For a while, I had two patients to check on during my visits, and Jethro progressed very well. He died some years after this incident. My patient kept his ashes on his bookcase as a reminder of this great dog.

Jethro was not the only furry creature I had to minister to. I had a ninety-year-old patient who lived in an apartment with her seventy-year-old daughter. Their calico cat, Princess, was a regal and loyal cat who followed my patient everywhere, even to the bathroom. One day when I made my monthly visit to give her a vitamin B12 injection, I found both her and her daughter distraught. There was something terribly wrong with Princess, who was hiding under the bed in the spare bedroom and wouldn't come out. They asked me to see what I could do. Now, I love cats—I had two cats growing up and am especially fond of calicoes—but I'm no cat whisperer. After taking care of my patient, I got down on the floor and peered under the bed at a growling, wide-eyed, crazed Princess. I could not get ahold of her and was at a loss as to how I could help.

I called the local vet, who was new in town, and he agreed to make a home visit. He arrived with a cat carrier and leather gloves and attempted to scare her out from under the bed. Princess was out like a shot and ran right up the door. I'd never seen a cat go vertical before. The vet was able to grab her and get her into the carrier and back to his office.

On my next visit, I was surprised to learn that Princess was still at the vet's. It seems that when the daughter cleaned the bathroom toilet, some bleach water had dripped from the toilet brush onto the floor, and

Princess had licked it up and scalded her throat. The vet had to anesthetize her and coat her throat with Maalox until she healed. She did get better, and came home to her relieved owners.

Unlike furry dogs and cats, which are easy to adjust to, other pets are more problematic. I like birds, for example, outside in the trees where they belong. So-called domesticated birds have caused me a few anxious moments.

I visited an elderly couple living in a cute little bungalow on a small farm in the country to give them their flu vaccines. The wife was in the kitchen and got her shot first. I then asked where her husband was, and she told me to go on down to the barn, where he was working in his wood shop. I proceeded to do just that. When I entered the barn, I was startled by a rustle above me. Looking up at the rafters, I saw a rooster flying at me with a vengeance. Let me tell you, I had no idea I could run that fast at thirty-five years of age. I ran out the side door of the barn, through the backyard, and into the side door of the house with that attack rooster only three steps behind me the whole way. I hate to think what would have happened if he'd caught me! He was a nasty fellow!

When I reentered the house, panting, the farmer's wife asked, "What's wrong?" I explained that a rooster had attempted to attack me. She calmly replied, "Oh, I forgot to tell you to take a stick from the porch before you go to the barn. That rooster is mean." I thought, "No kidding! Thanks for the information now, when it's a bit late."

When the farmer came up to the house from the woodshop (I wasn't going back, stick or no stick), I gave him his shot and asked him, "What's up with that rooster?" He told me that he had kept the rooster and other chickens in a pen by the river when they were young. Minks had come up from the river and killed all of them except this one rooster, which had been mean ever since. Clearly this couple had adapted to this survivor's trauma, taking a stick whenever they went to the barn. Personally, I wouldn't have been so charitable. But since my assigned area was changed shortly after this incident, I didn't have to deal with this attack rooster again, thank goodness!

Dickey Bird was a parakeet who lived with an elderly couple in a senior citizen apartment complex. They were very comfortable with him, allowing him to fly all over their home. But Dickey made me nervous; I was worried he'd land on me or, heaven forbid, poop on me. So I would call before my visit so that my patient could confine him to his cage.

One day, I arrived at their home, relieved to see Dickey safely locked away, but noticed something odd about the apartment. The pictures and mirrors had been turned around, and the stainless steel range hood had been covered with a garbage bag. When I asked my patient about these changes, she told me that Dickey Bird had started flying around, vomiting on anything that was shiny and reflective.

When I returned two weeks later, Dickey was in his cage and the apartment was back to normal. I asked if Dickey had stopped the vomiting behavior, and she said yes, the vet had told her that Dickey was lonesome, vomiting on his reflection to compensate for being alone. The solution: A plastic bird was put in the cage to keep him company. It worked. Dickey was happy to have a friend, I was happy that Dickey was in his cage, and the patient was happy that Dickey could again fly around without vomiting. Who knew that birds could get lonesome?

Parakeets can be a nuisance, but they're nothing compared to large, green jungle-size parrots. These birds are downright scary. They are *huge* and messy and can live to be more than one hundred years old.

I had a patient who kept her parrot in his own bedroom, which was a dull gray with no furniture in it; instead, it had a large tree branch where the parrot perched. There were newspapers all over the floor to catch his droppings, and the smell was atrocious.

One day, after she gave her pet a shower in the bathroom, he refused to go back to his room, and bit her on her upper breast, taking out a chunk of flesh one and a half inches deep. Due to the location of the wound, the patient was hesitant to tell her physician. Without the proper treatment, it had become infected, forcing her to go to the doctor. This is where I came into the picture. The doctor ordered daily wound irrigations with gauze packing, covered with a gauze pad. The location was such that the patient could not perform the dressing care herself, so I visited her daily for about two weeks. Fortunately, the wound healed well, and the parrot continued to live a nice long life in his bedroom without me!

I made a visit to a home that was not in great condition. Many windows were broken, there were no screens, and the walls had faded to some nondescript color. A neighbor had called because she had not seen the elderly gentleman who lived there in quite a while and wondered if he was all right.

When I knocked, a young man answered. I told him the reason for my visit and asked to see his father. The man ushered me in, telling me that his dad had not been to a doctor in years and lately had been unable to get out of bed. Over in the corner of the living room was a small twin bed pushed up against the wall where the withered, little man was lying. Everything was gray—his hair, his skin, even the sheets. He was really in poor condition. After I assessed the patient, he and the young man agreed that he would go to the ER to be evaluated. As I turned away from the patient, something suddenly flew right at me. It was a *huge* pigeon. It scared the daylights out of me! I thought, What's a pigeon doing inside the house? Then I looked around again, noticing the broken windows and open spaces, inviting critters inside.

As we waited for the ambulance, I tactfully suggested that maybe the windows should be repaired or at least the screens replaced so that pigeons would remain outside, where they belong—not flying at a person like a 747 jumbo jet inside the house. Needless to say, I was relieved when my patient left for the ER and I could fly the pigeon coop myself.

Not every bird is a scary, attacking, vomiting, biting, kamikaze pest. Occasionally, I could see the appeal.

One time, I went to see a patient in order to teach him how to use his new glucometer to check his blood sugar. When I entered his home, I noticed some birds in cages in his entry hall, but I really didn't pay much attention to them as we made our way back to the kitchen.

We sat at the kitchen table and went through all the glucometer instructions, step by step. When I finished and got ready to leave, I heard my voice saying, "Okay, okay, okay"—but I wasn't talking. One of the birds had obviously heard every word I said and sounded in voice and inflection exactly like me. I was astonished. He also made me realize that I say "okay" a lot. I'm no ornithologist, but I believe this clever fellow was a mynah bird. They're the ones that talk, right? Now, that is one bird I found to be quite entertaining.

Another time, when I was covering for a nurse who had called in sick, I visited a lady recovering from pneumonia who lived in a trailer. To assess the patient's cardiorespiratory status, I bent over to listen to her lung sounds, saying, "Now take a deep breath." Suddenly, something landed on my back. I must have jumped a mile, startling both the patient and the little lovebird, who apparently had seen my back as a landing strip. When I jumped, the bird quickly flew up to perch on top of the door. After I calmed down, the patient and I had a good laugh about the incident. She told me that this little mischief maker would frequently land on her shoulder or back and undo her necklaces. I was thankful that I hadn't harmed the bird in my reaction to her unscheduled landing. Once I got over the surprise, I found the little bird to be pretty and cute. But why people let a bird fly about in the house, I'll never understand.

This elderly gentleman lived with his wife in a small hamlet that was zoned for some farm animals. His home was very small: kitchen, front room, two bedrooms, and a bath. He was not feeling well, was extremely weak, and wasn't eating. Since he refused to go to the doctor, the family called the agency and asked for a home visit.

However, he didn't believe much in doctors and was pretty stubborn. But he had been a good friend of my grandfather's and let me examine him. He was not well, and I convinced him to go to the ER to be seen by a doctor since I needed a doctor's orders before I could provide home care. The patient was malnourished, constipated, and dehydrated. IV therapy perked him up, and the doctor ordered a specific diet and medication regimen and sent him home.

I went to the house to teach his wife about correct medication and fluid intake. Over the next few weeks, he improved quite a bit. He was walking, eating, drinking fluids, and following the doctor's orders. With his improved health, he began farming again.

On my next visit, I arrived to find him in the kitchen with two large cardboard boxes. In one box were three baby peacocks and in the other were three baby ostriches. Needless to say, I was not thrilled to see six birds in this tiny house, knowing that they would not stay small for long.

On my next visit, a couple of weeks later, I noticed the boxes in the kitchen were gone. When I inquired about the birds, he told me to open the second bedroom door. The room was divided by a wooden barrier, with peacocks on one side and four-foot-tall ostriches on the other. I closed the door quickly and asked, "What are you going to do with them?" He had made arrangements to sell them as soon as they were too big for the house. Why he had bought them in the first place was a mystery to me. Maybe once he started improving, he needed a project to engage him and give him a sense of accomplishment.

He was never short of ideas. Not all of them were well thought out. When it was nearing time to discharge him from our services, as he was much recovered, I made a visit to assess him and review his meds. When I arrived, I found the woodstove in pieces on the floor. I asked him why, and he told me that he was in the process of converting it to propane, because using the woodstove was becoming too difficult for his wife and him. I asked him, "Is that safe?" His less-than-reassuring response was, "Well, I'll make it work."

When I left, I made a beeline for the fire department. They knew him well and commented that if anyone could make it work, he could. Still, they agreed that it was not safe, so they made a home visit and talked him out of the conversion.

Then I met a bear! I had received a referral for a postoperative visit for a young man in his thirties who had had open-heart surgery. When I arrived, I did the usual paperwork, obtained his history, and then washed my hands to perform the physical assessment.

I took his blood pressure, temperature, and pulse, then asked him to open his shirt for me to assess his chest incision. At first glance, something looked odd. There was a clear adhesive dressing in place, the incision was aligned, and some bruising was present—all normal, except that his entire chest was also dark in color.

Upon further inspection, I finally understood what I was seeing. There was a large bear in the standing position tattooed on his chest. Its head was located just below his upper sternum, and the body extended down to his mid-abdomen. The bear's upper paws were spread open to the right and left of the body itself, with the legs standing together. The picture was so detailed, I could see every strand of fuzzy hair on the entire bear's body. That bear looked like it was ready to charge!

Of course, I had to ask the patient, "Is that an entire grizzly bear I'm seeing on your chest?" He answered yes, and explained that he had had a long talk with his surgeon after he learned he needed open-heart surgery and insisted the doctor not mess up his beautiful bear tattoo. That tattoo seemed more important to the patient than his cardiac condition!

The surgeon certainly did a fabulous job—the image of that bear was perfectly intact. The chest incision was cut right down the middle of the bear, and the surgeon had realigned every tattooed hair. The edges of the incision were flawlessly stapled together, and it was as straight as an arrow. I was really quite impressed and amazed. The patient commented, "He cut right on the dotted line."

Now I had to change that Tegaderm dressing. This particular type of dressing adheres to the skin very well, and the best way to remove it is to loosen a corner, apply light pressure, and pull it away from the skin. It can be mildly uncomfortable but shouldn't be extremely painful. I began the removal, and you would have thought I was cutting my patient with a knife. He started yelling, "OH!!! AH!!! SHIT!!! That's killing me!"

Of course I stopped, let him rest, and then proceeded extremely slowly, finally getting the old dressing off. I cleansed the incision with sterile water and gauze and applied the new dressing.

I could not help myself. I had to ask him. "How painful was it to have that huge detailed grizzly bear tattooed on your chest? It certainly had to hurt more than that dressing removal." His response was, surprisingly, "Not bad."

He really was a nice guy, but he did seem to have a low threshold for pain. In the end, he recovered well, and at the time of discharge from our agency, his nicely healed bear tattoo on his chest was looking just fine.

Being more of a city gal myself, encounters with farm animals could be frightening—like the aforementioned attack rooster—or enlightening, like the horses on this lovely lady's large horse farm.

I know nothing about horses, and they seem to detect that about me. Frankly, they scare me. One day as I was concluding my medical visit with this patient, her daughter came up from the barn and her mother asked, "Have you lifted her yet?" The question was in reference to a new foal that had been born a few weeks earlier. When I asked her what she was talking about, she explained that when a foal is small, it has to be raised so that all four hooves are off the ground. Though this scares the foal a bit, it also establishes who is in charge, making it easier to train the horse and gain its respect. What an interesting, heretofore unknown piece of information!

When I visited this patient a few weeks later, I learned something else about horses. It was a beautiful spring day and happened to be her birthday. She was sitting in her wheelchair on the front porch, enjoying the pleasant weather. I had pulled up a chair beside her and started taking her blood pressure, when I spotted her daughter coming up from the barn with my patient's beautiful one-thousand-pound horse named Baby Dawn in tow. When the animal reached the porch edge, she gently climbed the two steps and laid her head right in my patient's lap, allowing her to stroke Baby Dawn's soft nose and enjoy her company. It was a beautiful moment, showing the profound, loving bond these two had. I'd never seen anything like it and was deeply moved witnessing their connection.

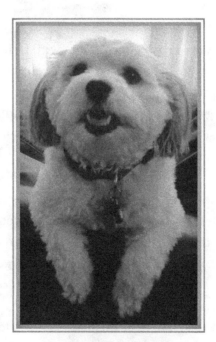

MY SISTER'S DOG, JETER.

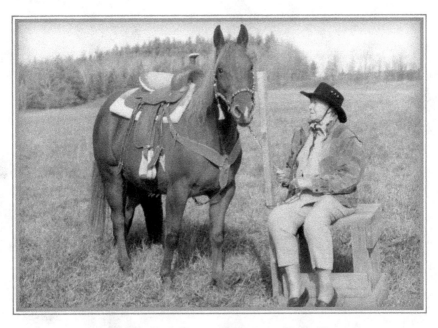

MY DEAR PATIENT WITH HER HORSE, BABY DAWN.
THE PHOTO WAS A CHRISTMAS PRESENT TO ME FROM HER FAMILY
IN DECEMBER 1999.

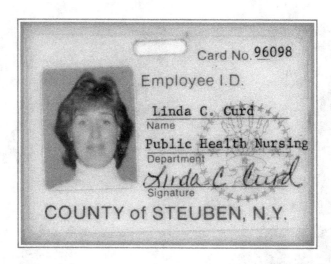

My nursing ID badge from work, mid-1980s.

FOUR

DIFFERENT STROKES

Learn the dance. Determine how to tactfully assert your authority in someone else's space while being respectful. Dealing with others' cultures and lifestyles may prove challenging.

SINCE PUBLIC HEALTH nurses work on patients in their homes, it can be difficult to be both a respectful guest and, at the same time, a professional caregiver. Our job requires proficiency at our various tasks and a level of cleanliness that not every home has. It's always a hard call when your own personal thoughts and judgment clash with the client's or their family caregiver. I've prayed with patients and their families. I've respected the differences in their cultures compared to mine. I did my best to be prepared for challenges that could affect my ability to do the job, but there were times when something unexpected occurred, and I had to quickly determine the best way to be respectful while still doing my job.

Oftentimes, bedrooms are not easily accessible or large enough to accommodate hospital equipment and beds. Consequently, the bed and the patient might be placed in one of the larger, more public rooms of the home, such as a living room or dining room. When I first started making home visits, that wasn't much of an issue. Though there weren't doors or curtains, during the day there was still a measure of privacy while family members were at school or work, and I was able to perform personalized care without breaching the patient's privacy. I rarely ran into any school-aged children except in the summer. This really changed in the late 1980s and '90s, when homeschooling became more popular. Once schoolchildren entered the equation, I had to find a way to make nursing care more discreet.

I was in one home taking care of the homeowner's elderly mother, who had to have her catheter changed monthly. On this particular visit, she had her ten-year-old grandson there. Her hospital bed was in the open dining room, with no way to shut doors or pull curtains in order to seclude her from the adjacent rooms. I mentioned that we needed to change her catheter and suggested that maybe the grandson might like to go outside or upstairs for about twenty to thirty minutes while I performed the procedure. His mother said to me, "Oh no, he wants to be a doctor, so I think it would be educational if he watched." This really took me aback. I certainly did not agree with that at all, but unfortunately, the grandmother was too infirm to express her opinion on the matter. I had to come up with a tactful way to protect the patient's privacy without offending the mother or causing her son to act up. Finally, I said, "This is a sterile procedure, and I don't think it's appropriate for a ten-year-old boy to observe his grandmother getting catheterized." That got the desired result without further discussion. However, I really wonder what that mother could possibly have been thinking.

Sometimes, the hardest issue to resolve is what constitutes appropriate versus offensive behavior. I had this lovely young woman as a patient who had had a cerebral aneurysm. Her surgery to repair/remove the aneurysm was successful, but after surgery, she suffered a mild bleed, leaving her paralyzed on the right side. I called ahead to tell her I was coming for a post-op visit to assess her vitals and review her meds. When I got to her home I found the door open—not unusual, since with her paralysis, it was difficult for her to get to the door quickly. I walked in and yelled her name—also not unusual. She responded, "I'm back here in the bedroom." I went down the hall and found her in bed, again not unusual. However, what was unusual is that her boyfriend was in bed with her. And both were naked. Here I am in my uniform, bag on my shoulder, ready to do an assessment, in a situation that I found totally embarrassing. She thought nothing of it and said, "Don't worry about it. You can go ahead and do what you need to do. We don't mind."

I have to say, that was the first and only time I did a nursing assessment, sitting on the portable toilet next to the bed, with the patient and her boyfriend both naked in bed. Though it wasn't comfortable, I made the best of it, doing what I had come there to do. They didn't seem bothered in the least. For me, I was grateful he didn't get out of bed in front of me!

It's not always easy to know what to do in a given situation. In this case, their level of comfort with the situation was far greater than mine. I didn't want to offend, cause a scene, have to reschedule, or insist that my naked, paralyzed patient move to a location that was more private. Was that the right call? I don't know. After that, whenever I needed to visit her, I called ahead as usual, but also asked if she could be out of bed before I arrived.

What I tried to remember in every visit is that I am a guest in my patients' homes. Unless what they are doing is a danger to themselves or others, what they do and how they act in their own homes is their business. Fortunately, most folks are kind, considerate, and grateful to have a nurse visit to provide care.

Migrant workers came north to our county at the end of summer through early fall, mainly to harvest the potato fields. This was before the automated potato harvester. Most of the workers went back down to Georgia and the Carolinas after the potato harvest here. They hated the cold and were eager to get back to the South, where there was warm weather and more crops to pick.

But there was a camp where some migrants did stay year-round, and that's mainly where I visited those who needed care. I was in my twenties, naive and ignorant about their lives and their lifestyle. The camp was made up of older-style trailers dispersed throughout the grounds, and two cement barracks, each containing about ten one-room apartments. What always caught my eye was the outhouse/shower facilities. It was a cinder block building with a separation: MEN painted on the blocks on the right side, and WO-MEN painted on the left side.

My first visit with a patient typically began with the recording of personal details: date of birth, place of birth, and address. I was shocked that so many did not know these details beyond their names, which often were those of famous historical personages such as George Washington, Thomas Jefferson, and Robert E. Lee. In addition to not knowing the details of their birth, the workers often did not know who their fathers were, what the names of their siblings were, and sometimes, even how old they were. The concept of someone not knowing these details about his or her life was foreign to me.

Though getting details was somewhat difficult, I was pleased that, for the most part, the workers cooperated. One theory regarding this cooperation was that they respected our uniforms. In my case, though, it was more likely the support I had from their six-foot-three-inch, two-hundred-and-seventy-five-pound, extremely handsome crew chief with a chiseled face and square jaw. His arms were so muscular, it was difficult to make the standard blood pressure cuff fit.

One day, the crew chief asked me to listen to his lungs. I heard a dull sound in one quadrant and told him to see the doctor. He was diagnosed with lung cancer. As a result of this early detection, he lived another five years and credited me with prolonging his life. Out of gratitude and respect, he made it a point to look out for me when I was at the camp. After he passed away, his son was not as protective of me, and I didn't feel as safe.

His son did not have his father's looks, impressive size, or the respect of the migrant workers. He was lazy and definitely lacked leadership skills. Consequently, the camp fell apart. If I had to return to the camp during that time, I was advised to go with a second person. Even the state troopers went in pairs if they were called. And they were armed.

One important part of our work as public health nurses was to routinely test the workers for possible active tuberculosis. Upon arriving at camp, we would have the workers line up and attempt to get their personal details, obtain a signed permission form (this was a bit challenging, as many were illiterate), and perform the Mantoux skin test, which involved injecting the patient with a serum intradermally, waiting forty-eight to seventy-two hours, and going back to check for a reaction.

Three days after the skin test, we would go back to the camp to read the results. We always hoped it wasn't raining, as rain meant there would be no work that day, and the workers would be drunk or difficult to find. They would drink anything with alcohol in it, including shoe polish, Aqua Velva aftershave, even rubbing alcohol mixed with RC Cola. Boredom and isolation encouraged their drinking behavior.

In most of the cases, the results of the test would be positive, but not active for tuberculosis. The testing was to prevent tuberculosis infections from spreading up and down the East Coast. The migrants with the most positive of tests would be treated and followed if they left the area. Frequently, my supervisor was in contact with the other home health agencies along the migrants' routes south for follow-up, as they continued to follow the crop harvest. If someone was symptomatic, showing respiratory symptoms, he or she would receive a chest X-ray and more follow-up. Those with very positive tests—including showing a large lump on the arm, redness (which was sometimes hard to detect), and warmth at the site—were treated with oral medication. Unfortunately, many were not good about taking these pills when they were supposed to. When we returned, I would count their pills to see if they were taking them correctly. Most of the time, I would leave a week's supply of fourteen pills—one pill to be taken twice a day—then return in a week and count twelve pills still in the bottle. Not a good sign!

One day a colleague and I were searching for a fellow who had missed his readings. When I asked about his whereabouts, I was told he was down in the "bull pen," a building away from the barracks. We walked right down there and opened the door on a group of men. We asked to see him to read his skin test, and all of a sudden the place became very quiet. The men slowly got up and surrounded us. There we were: two nonthreatening women trying to do our jobs, not looking for any trouble, facing a wall of hardened men. It was midday, but very dark in the bull pen. Literally all we could see were the whites of their eyes. The hair stood up on the back of my neck. Was there a fluttering of panic in me? Without question! We bolted out of there. Later I learned that the bull pen was for men only. No women—especially white women—

were allowed. We were lucky to get out of there in one piece. Needless to say, we never did get that man's reading.

A few migrant workers I met in the seventies became lifetime patients. When I first met M, I was shocked that she had no eyes. I knocked on her trailer door at the migrant camp to perform a skin test, and when she answered, all I saw were two red, empty eye sockets. I was startled, to say the least. Thankfully, she could not see the astonished look on my face. I later heard a rumor that M's lesbian lover had torn her eyes out in a jealous rage when she looked at another woman. I noticed scarring around M's empty eye sockets, making me wonder briefly if the story might be true. However, she had suffered from diabetes for a long time, which was more likely the cause of the missing eyes. The rumor was probably just that—a rumor.

Years later, M was living in an adult rest home and was able to obtain prosthetic eyes. I received another referral to see her and teach her how to use a talking glucometer. Being independent with the glucometer meant that she could stay at the rest home. One day during my visit with her, I complimented her on her pretty red dress. She was livid. She said, "Red? I'm wearing red? I HATE RED!" She didn't know what color she was wearing until I told her. If I'd known, I wouldn't have said a word! I continued to follow her for many years and we became dear friends.

Another female migrant worker who shocked me on my first meeting, but for an entirely different reason, was ML, a six-foot-tall woman with hands so large she could palm a basketball. Her hair was wild, standing straight up all over her head like a crazed lion. I went to the barracks to assess her partner, R, the only white man in the camp. ML answered the door, looked me up and down, and told me in no uncertain terms that if I looked at R in a "special way," she would kill me! I believed her!

From that inauspicious beginning came a long professional relationship with ML and R. From time to time over the years, both were patients requiring the services of public health nursing. One incident involved my treating R when he pulled out his catheter after prostate removal. He was frustrated with that tube, as he couldn't have sex with ML, so he pulled it out. With some force, I might add. After I stabilized him, I called his urologist who said that as long as he could urinate and he was not bleeding, the catheter could be left out. He was seeing his doctor the next day, so my job was done.

However, as I prepared to leave, I noticed that ML did not appear to be all right. There was no alcohol on her breath, which was unusual, and her blood pressure was very low. Her blood sugar was in range, but her eyes were rolling back in her head. As there was no phone in the house, I used my newly purchased cell phone to call the hospital. She had no current doctor, so I felt she needed to go to the ER. I got permission from the hospital social worker to send her there and called the ambulance, giving all the information I had to the drivers.

She arrived at the hospital nearly comatose. A CT scan revealed a subdural hematoma. Later, I learned that earlier in the week, she had fallen off her back porch railing and hit the back of her head, apparently resulting in a slow bleed in her brain. Thankfully, because I had been at her home and noticed her behavior changes, the hematoma was discovered in time to prevent any permanent damage, and she received the treatment she needed. After three weeks in rehabilitation, she returned home.

One rewarding aspect of being a public health nurse was these relationships I forged with unlikely people. Who could have predicted that M, with the "torn out" eyes, and ML, who had threatened to kill me, would become cherished patients and friends? When ML passed away, the obituary had few details, saying she had "no known relatives." A reporter from the local paper was struck by that and decided to follow up with a longer article, in which he described ML as a "tall woman from the [Mississippi] Delta who spent most of her adult life crouched over, in fields, dying without family and buried in a hillside in the Southern Tier of Western New York." He also attended the funeral and was gratified that, although she didn't have any known family, she was rich in friends, including one from her Delta days. The minister, quoted in the article, said, "Although [ML's] relatives were not known, she had friends, and she had people who cared about her. . . . To have friends makes you wealthy indeed." I was still following M at the time of ML's passing, so I cut out that article and read it to M. She was so grateful to learn what had happened to her friend from the migrant camps.

In our county's rural areas, we have quite a large community of Amish families. The Amish avoid modern technology and transportation because they view it as a connection to the outside world, a world filled with temptations that can destroy the all-important family and community. As a result, their homes have no electricity, no indoor plumbing except a pump in the kitchen for cold water, and no telephones. To get from one place to another, they rely on horse and buggies or on someone outside the community to drive them in cars. For the most part, they keep to themselves, relying on one another to meet their needs. Occasionally, however, they require assistance from those outside their community. Providing nursing care in this different environment can be challenging.

I received a referral on an eleven-year-old Amish boy who had taken a serious fall in his barn. He spent weeks in the hospital while his many internal injuries were stabilized. In addition, he had fractured his leg in several places. When he returned home, his leg was encased in a metal apparatus that was pinned in four places to his leg. My job was to perform the pin care at first, eventually instructing his family on how to do that, and assess his overall healing.

When I arrived at his home, I was greeted by the boy's many siblings—about ten, I believe—and his father. His mother had died in a car accident a few months before the boy's fall. She had gone with about six other Amish folks to visit a hydroponic farm about forty-five miles away in a neighbor's van. The van was sideswiped at an intersection, and the Amish ladies in the back were killed in the crash. It was a real tragedy for the entire community.

One would expect, with so many children, that the house would be noisy and chaotic. However, the home was orderly, sparsely furnished, simple, and very clean. The boy's father and older sisters ran the household. The family communicated quietly in German with one another and in English with me.

My patient was the cutest little boy, with long blond curls and the most beautiful clear green eyes. In addition, he had a cute yellow parakeet. As you know, I don't much care for feathered creatures, but this young boy and his pet made a charming duo. The boy would give a quick whistle and the little bird would come land on his shoulder.

My patient was lovable and so very brave. He never complained, even though I could tell that I was hurting him as I cleaned around the pin sites. He was determined to get well. After a few weeks, he figured out a way to get himself out of bed without help and move around with a walker without applying weight on his leg. His agility with that metal apparatus was amazing. It was obvious that this family really took care of each other. His older sisters, who made all the clothes for the family, made adjustments to his trousers by opening the seam and applying ties so that he could wear his pants but still have the pin sites accessible for care.

I eventually taught his sisters standard pin care, which required that each pin be cleaned with a sterile Q-tip dipped in a mix of half peroxide and half saline, covered with a split two-by-two-inch gauze dressing, and secured with tape. It was fortunate that the hospital mailed his supplies right to the house, because we went through so many dressings and Q-tips with each treatment. When I would call the hospital from my cell phone to reorder supplies, the nurses would always ask how he was doing. I believe he left a lasting impression on them also.

Circumstances were such that I was unable to continue caring for this little Amish boy. His father explained to me that the hospital bills were enormous, and even with the assistance of their community, they were in financial straits and didn't have the money to continue treatment. Since the Amish would not take government benefits, he needed to find an alternative. The boy's grandfather had a home in Massachusetts near a Shriners hospital, and he was being sent there, where he would still be with family and receive free medical care. I was sad to see him go, but I understood the financial necessity.

I was taken by this family, so loving to one another and so committed to their values and way of life. Their ability to use their hands to farm, to make clothes, to cook and preserve food, and to build beautiful furniture was so impressive. On one of my last visits to the home I walked into the dining room and saw a gorgeous six-foot-tall cherry dresser. One of the older brothers had made it as a wedding gift for his oldest sister. What an act of love!

I've always wondered how my little patient fared after he left. I want to believe that he healed well and has lived a long, happy life.

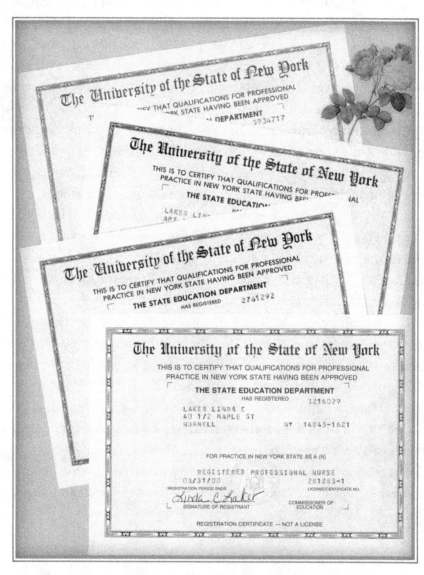

ALL MY PAST NEW YORK STATE NURSING LICENSES.

FIVE

DANGERS

Be aware, and as much as possible,
be prepared for the possibility of danger.

WORKING IN A mainly rural area, there were not many times when I felt threatened, but there were a few. As I've shared, animals can be defensive and unpredictable. And there were also those couple of moments with the migrant workers when a situation could have turned violent, but did not—thank goodness. Aside from those, there was one other precarious incident I'll never forget.

I had a volatile and emotional Italian woman as a client. On this particular day, she had been served divorce papers from her husband and totally lost control of her emotions. She was suicidal, threatening to use natural gas to blow up her home and herself, at the same time endangering her neighbors. She was about two weeks postoperative from a knee replacement, so her mobility was compromised. Her social worker asked if I'd come and talk with her along with one of the nuns from the church to see if we could calm her down. When we got to her home, she let us in but was clearly in distress, limping about restlessly like a caged animal. Alarmed, I called the psychiatrist, who instructed me not to talk to her or engage her anymore, but instead to call an ambulance, and he would commit her to the psychiatric ward in the hospital.

The situation was tricky. Here I am, in the kitchen with a frail and elderly five-foot-two, ninety-pound nun, waiting for the ambulance while the patient is in the other room ranting and raving. Then things got worse. Hearing the commotion, the neighbors called the police, who arrived at the house before the ambulance. My patient rushed into the kitchen, grabbed a steak knife, and tried to stab me. I was shocked! I had never been physically assaulted before, and I immediately went into action, totally forgetting about her knee. I quickly slammed her up against the counter, took away the knife, and pushed her into a chair. The poor nun was as white as a sheet. I needed to act defensively to protect myself and potentially anyone else if she had retained the knife.

That was the first round. The danger wasn't over. As one policeman walked by the woman's chair, she tried to grab his gun. Not only was I nearly stabbed, but I could have been shot as well. The policeman clearly wasn't much help controlling the situation. He then had the poor judgment to ask me to take her into the bathroom, alone, because she wanted to change her clothes before going to the hospital. I said to him, "Are you kidding me? She just tried to stab me and then shoot me. I'm not taking her anywhere!"

When the ambulance finally arrived, my favorite fireman was the first one in the door. He is a large but gentle man, six foot two, two hundred and fifty pounds, and a no-nonsense kind of guy. I graduated from high school with his brother, so we knew each other well. I proceeded to fill him in and give him the details he needed: "She's dangerous! The psychiatrist at the hospital is aware of the situation and is planning to commit her. I want you to pick her up and strap her down on the gurney." He did exactly that, no questions asked. I was never so relieved in my life.

When the psychiatrist heard the details of the situation, he called and asked to see me in his office. He was so kind, wanting to make sure that I hadn't been traumatized by the events. I was shaken up but okay. After talking to my supervisor, the police, and the psychiatrist, I went home, where I finally started to cry. It was a delayed reaction and a necessary release. I was so relieved that neither I nor anyone else had been hurt. I truly believe someone was watching over me that day.

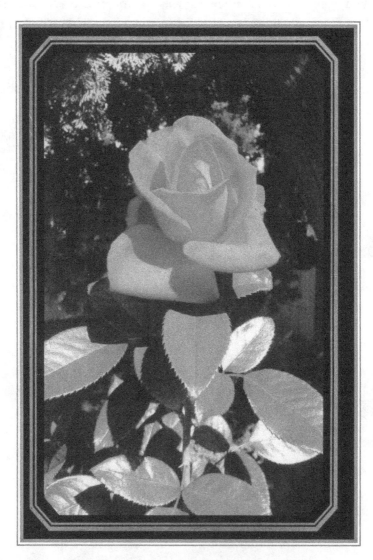

A MISTER LINCOLN ROSE FROM MY GARDEN.

SIX

CAREGIVERS

Caregivers are often a crucial part of patient care.

CAREGIVERS ARE BEST described as those who take care of another in need, be it a spouse or a family member or friend; in the case of home care, we are caregivers to strangers who become our patients. I never could have done my job without the dedicated home health aides and family, friends, and partners who were willing to step up to the plate and learn some really skilled nursing procedures. It's ideal when the public health nurses, home health aides, and family members work together to provide for the patient at home.

Home health aides are the unsung heroes of home care. They are a special breed of caregiver who not only make sure the patient's personal care needs are met, but also perform household tasks. In a single day they would bathe and dress the patient, change the bed, start laundry, dust, mop the kitchen and bath, do the dishes, and possibly make a light lunch for the patient before leaving. These aides, usually women, might make as many as five visits in a day before going home to care for their own families.

Many times I needed a home health aide's assistance when caring for a patient, for tasks that required another pair of hands. When necessary, I'd schedule my visits to coincide with the home health aide's so that she could assist me in positioning a patient, opening a package after I had put on my sterile gloves, or helping with a complex procedure, such as a dressing change or catheter insertion. Their assistance was invaluable to me.

I appreciated and respected them and never wanted to take them for granted. If my visit to a patient occurred while the home health aide was working, I would frequently jump in to help with bathing the patient or changing the bed. In addition, I felt strongly that I should never ask an aide to do something I wasn't willing to do myself, including some of the less pleasant tasks: emptying commodes, catheter bags, or bed pans.

An example that has stayed with me over the years involves a patient who was paralyzed from the waist down. To describe him as difficult and demanding would be an understatement. He was angry at the world. He was the type of person who wrote scathing editorials in the newspaper complaining about everybody and everything, or called into the hometown radio show to complain about the local government and employees. He was never satisfied. He lived alone in a trailer that was spotless. His carpet was stark white—you'll understand why I include that fact in a minute. When you were in his home, everything had to be just so: perfectly in order and immaculate.

Every morning the agency's home health aide performed his personal care, helped him dress, and transferred him to his wheelchair using a Hoyer lift. On one particular day, he was suffering from constipation and needed an enema. I connected with the home health aide because I required her assistance to perform this procedure. We finished the upper part of his bath, then I administered a Fleet enema. In those days, we could perform that procedure without the use of gloves, just good clean hands. We rolled him to his right side and then over to the left, then placed him in the Hoyer lift sling, and proceeded to transfer him from his bed to the commode; the lift sling has a hole in the bottom for this purpose. As he was in midair, about three feet from the commode, he started to yell, "Hurry, hurry, hurry! I'm going!" The home health aide and I were moving him as fast as we could, when suddenly . . . he went. In a split second, I held out my hand and caught the mess. Disaster averted. The dumbfounded home health aide maneuvered him onto the pot and commented, "I can't believe you just did that," as I made my way to the bathroom to wash my hands—about ten times, I might add. Thank goodness for lots of soap and hot water.

It was a split-second decision, but one I didn't regret for an instant. If that stark white carpet had been stained, we would never have heard the end of it. He would have made our lives more miserable than he already was. That sweet home health aide was my friend for life. She went on to school to become a registered nurse, and we laughed about that day for many years to come.

When multiple home-care services are provided, the average time for a home health aide visit can be anywhere from thirty minutes up to three hours, depending on the patient's needs. Conversely, most of my visits were twenty to thirty minutes long, unless I had a complicated procedure to perform.

I had a sweet gentleman patient, a widower in his late eighties, who lived in the country. I visited him every other week, once to administer his B12, the second to supervise the home health aide. In this case, the home health aide visited him for one to two hours three times a week to assist with showering, dressing, laundry, light housekeeping, and dishes. Since he received deliveries from Meals on Wheels, food preparation was minimal.

One day on a visit near Christmas, I found the home health aide making him lunch. As a Christmas present, she had bought him a dozen eggs and made him an apple pie with Splenda, since he was diabetic. He was thrilled to have two fried eggs with toast and apple pie for dessert. It hadn't occurred to me that after getting prepared meals for years, he would appreciate a home-cooked meal, but the home health aide knew. This was such a treat for him. That was just one act of kindness out of the many I observed from the wonderful home health aides I worked with.

The year I retired from public health nursing, a luncheon for all those who were retiring—two supervisors and me—was held. When I walked into the banquet hall, my heart was warmed by the presence of the home health aides whom I had worked with over the years. They all came, each with their special signature dish to pass. I was so surprised and humbled. I could never have done my job and looked after so many folks without their assistance. It was truly a special moment, and I'll never forget the hard-working, caring home health aides of our agency.

Aside from the home health aides, there have been a few memorable family caregivers over the years. We taught laypeople how to give injections, perform colostomy care, help the patient self-catheterize, use sterile dressing techniques, administer IV therapy, perform gastrostomy tube feeding, and much more. Some took to it quickly, while others took some encouragement, saying, "I never wanted to be a nurse." I'd reply, "Well you've got to learn. I can only make so many visits and can't be here 24/7. So, here we go." Oftentimes, the caregivers made as much of an impression on me as the patient.

H and C were a wonderful couple. C was a beautiful, artistic lady from Germany—I loved her accent—who had a bedroom converted into her art studio. Her works were mostly lovely still life paintings. H, my patient, was a retired chemical engineer who had worked for Corning Glass. Theirs was a true love story. They met when H attended a conference for work in Toronto, at a hotel where C, a German immigrant, was working banquets and high-end conferences. They fell in love, and she joined him in the States to begin their life together.

I met this couple when C asked H's doctor for a referral and home assessment after he had suffered a series of minor strokes. He had difficulty with ambulation and daily activities, so part of my job was to evaluate his physical therapy needs. This would be followed up by a visit from a physical therapist, who would set up an exercise program and instruct C on how to carry out the regimen. Another part of my job was to assess the home and see how it could be made safer, which also involved instructing C on how to help H in transfers (for example, getting in and out of bed or using the toilet) and in dressing and bathing. A home health aide was assigned to assist her in these tasks. She was a marvelous student, so willing to rearrange her home and do what was necessary to care for her spouse. You could tell how much they loved each other by their willingness to work together for his benefit.

On about my third visit to their home, I pulled into the driveway and found C in her exquisite rose garden. I had been thinking about planting a few roses in my own yard, so I asked her what the secret was to growing such fabulous flowers in zone five. She then asked me what my favorite rose is. I am rather particular when it comes to roses. Most roses available in florist shops have no odor because some people are allergic. But what is the first thing a person does when handed a bouquet of flowers? Smell them, of course. I told her, "Any red rose with a lovely scent." She recommended Mister Lincoln, a beautiful long-stem, deep-red rose with a fragrance that can fill a room. I hunted for Mister Lincoln roses and finally settled on Lasting Love, a Mister Lincoln hybrid.

I took great care in planting it in my garden. This beautiful bush blooms every June, coincidentally usually on my mother's birthday. Eventually, I found the Mister Lincoln rose in a catalogue, ordered it, and planted it behind the Lasting Love bush. Mister Lincoln produces gorgeous roses with a bloom that is sometimes four to five inches in diameter, and a scent that fills my home—just as C had said it would.

When my roses bloom, I always think of dear C, who shared her special knowledge of roses with me and who had such a fond and loving relationship with her dear husband, H. Sometimes folks pass through your life. It may be brief, but they leave a lasting memory. C and H were that kind of people. I give my roses to friends all summer long to share their beauty and the love I feel when I think of where my rose garden got its start.

V and J were another lovely, loving couple who actually were my neighbors. V was a retired high school English teacher, and J was a retired lawyer who had had his own private practice in town.

J had a CVA—cerebrovascular accident, commonly known as a stroke—leaving him paralyzed on his left side. He was a very tall, thin man, and V was short and stout. She loved her home and was determined to care for J there, but she did not want to make her home into a hospital, and she accomplished that.

V turned her dining room into a space to care for J. She even had an antique privacy screen by his bed. I made a home visit and gave V suggestions regarding where to place the hospital bed, commode, wheelchair, and all the needed equipment. J seemed very comfortable, and V was fine with upsetting her dining room.

At one of my next visits, J needed to use the commode, and I assisted V with his safe transfer. Then V went to the kitchen to make coffee. When J was done, I was looking feverishly for the toilet paper. I could not find it anywhere. V returned to the dining room and I asked, "Where is the toilet paper for J?" V said matter-of-factly, "It's in the ice bucket." She said it as if that was the most common place to have toilet paper! We all had a good laugh over that.

One day after I had assessed J and knew he was comfortable, V gave me a house tour. She and J had no children, so their home was set up for just the two of them. When we went upstairs, I noted V had taken a small bedroom and made it into her laundry room. She told me, "You create all your laundry upstairs, why have a laundry in the basement?" I remembered that when we renovated our own home. Our bedroom is on the third floor and so is my laundry. Thanks to V's hint, laundry is not a chore in my house.

On another visit to J, a Friday, it happened to be my birthday. Since V and J were my neighbors, they invited me to stop in after work for a drink. I gladly went, and we had a wonderful evening. They were truly an interesting couple, considering their classroom and legal experience, and I enjoyed them very much.

When J died, I went to the calling hours, and there sat V in a beautiful black dress with pearls. I told her how sad I was for her loss and complimented her on how lovely she looked. V then told me that this particular funeral parlor had been her childhood home where she grew up. I was amazed. Then she said, "I wore my pearls for J, as this is our last dance." I'll never forget that. V and J were two lovely people whom I had the privilege to get to know through my job. How wonderful!

R, a cute, funny, and clever little Irishman, was a widower who had COPD and required continuous oxygen, but who didn't let that slow him down much. When I first met him, he was sitting in his favorite chair, which he took with him whenever he changed locations. It was a brown- and beige-plaid overstuffed recliner with just the right wear patterns to fit his body. His oxygen tubing hung down his back, which was unusual; most folks have the cannula in their nose with the hose down the front. Well, that hose irritated him so much, he placed the cannula in his nose and ran the tubing down his back, with a safety pin securing it to his shirt. A rather ingenious way to keep the tubing out from under his feet!

He was tickled to find out that I'm Irish also and loved to chat with me and tell me stories. And I loved to listen. Frequently, I'd listen to his lungs first and then he could start his stories while I finished the rest of his assessment, checking ankle edema, weight, appetite, and bowels. I could often tell how well his lungs were working by how much conversation we could have without his becoming short of breath.

He loved the hustle and bustle of his family. His four daughters obviously loved him and came up with a unique plan for sharing the care of their dad. Each of them had a dedicated bedroom in their own homes for his three-month rotational visits. That way, no one got irritated with him or felt unfairly burdened with his care. For nine months of the calendar year, he was with the three daughters who lived out of my area. He was my patient when his rotation brought him to my neck of the woods during the months of March, April, and May.

Since he arrived in my area with Saint Patrick's Day around the corner, I sent him a card. Well, you'd think I'd given him a million dollars. He was very proud of his Irish roots, and was so thankful and thrilled that I had thought about him on St. Pat's. But, after all, how could I not?

I've never seen this much cooperation within a family. They were all ready and willing to care for their dad, and all of them immediately accepted the challenge of caring for him. He and his wife had clearly done something right in the raising of their daughters into loving, caring individuals. This sweet man and his devoted family touched my heart.

Caregivers provide assistance to their loved ones to the best of their abilities. They are involved in the patient's medical care and are largely responsible for everyday needs, such as personal care and food. This next example, however, takes food provision to a whole new level.

For some reason I've always designated this family as Wynken, Blynken, and Nod: Wynken, who was cleverer than he let on, and his two mentally challenged sisters, Blynken and Nod. The sisters were simple, but pleasant, and both diabetic. They lived in a remote area of the county. I don't believe Nod, the youngest, had ever been away from home except for one terrifying hospitalization. Being without the familiar comfort of home and family frightened her so. Our agency provided home health aides to assist with the sisters' personal care and nurses to monitor the diabetes. Wynken was the family caregiver/provider. We worked with this family for many, many years.

One morning I arrived at about 8:15 to check the sisters' fasting blood sugars and fill their insulin syringes, which Wynken would administer over the next two weeks. When I stepped into the kitchen, there was a noxious, foul odor, so bad I can't describe it. Wynken and Blynken were canning something. The pots were boiling away, and the two were stuffing some kind of food product into each canning jar. Once I was able to withstand the stench enough to form sentences, I asked what the food was. Blynken responded, "Deer meat." I commented to the brother, "I didn't know you went deer hunting anymore." Blynken's response floored me. "Oh, he doesn't. We picked it up off the side of the road yesterday on the way home from town."

I was struck dumb. What do I say or do next? It dawned on me that this probably was not the first time they had harvested roadkill for their meals. I also knew that I wasn't going to change their behavior. When I wrote up my report, I included my discovery and went on with my day. Over the several years our agency cared for them, they showed no ill effects from their roadside acquisitions. After my nursing area was changed to the southern part of the county, I lost track of the family, but later I learned that the Blynken and Nod had suffered strokes at different times and ended up in a skilled nursing facility, while Wynken continued to live on the farm until he passed.

SEVEN

SICK CHILDREN

*When dealing with young patients, extra tact
and emotional support are often required.*

IT IS ONE thing when an adult is injured or becomes ill. It is another
when the patient is a child. Adults, for the most part, comprehend
what's going on and can partake readily in their own care. When a
child is diagnosed with a major illness, it can be especially frightening.
I can't say enough about the children's hospitals that take care of these
sweet little kids with cancer. Whether it's St. Jude, Shriners, Golisano,
or Roswell, they are all wonderful and treat not only the child, but take
care of the families as well.

I would usually get a referral when the child was first diagnosed and
had come home with a catheter in his or her chest or some other device
or port that needed attention. The moms and dads were always taught
well and would do the sterile dressing changes. Our responsibility
would be blood draws from the catheter, emotional support, and general assessments of the patient. Those hospitals were only a phone call
away and always got right on the phone and answered any questions or
concerns we may have had at any given moment.

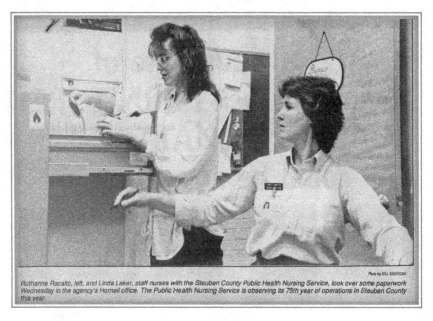

Ruthanne Racalto, left, and Linda Laker, staff nurses with the Steuben County Public Health Nursing Service, look over some paperwork Wednesday in the agency's Hornell office. The Public Health Nursing Service is observing its 75th year of operations in Steuben County this year.

ME AT MY DESK IN THE OFFICE, EARLY 1990S.

Three particular young patients stand out in my memory. I had to be especially sensitive to their emotional states in order to best help them cope with their serious illnesses. I grew very attached to these brave youngsters and hope they grew up healthy and happy after their difficult ordeals. Overall, I was fortunate that most of the children I cared for recovered and, as far as I know, did well.

I had a cute four-year-old girl patient with long, beautiful brown hair, who was the darling of the household. She had four older brothers; I think she was a surprise baby since her closest brother was twelve years older. She had been diagnosed with acute myeloid leukemia, and I was seeing her for weekly blood draws. The blood test results would dictate whether or not she could receive chemotherapy that week.

On one visit, I found her playing in her room, and when I asked her to come out for her assessment and blood draw, I noticed her dog. Clearly, the little girl had turned her older docile pet into her patient. Going into the extra supply bag, provided for her own care, she had secured an IV cap with an extension set to the back of her dog using Tegaderm dressing—a clear, plastic, and sticky dressing. When she came out of the bedroom with her dog bounding out right behind her, all I could see was the IV extension set and cap flopping in the air as he trotted into the room. I never laughed so hard as when I saw that wiener dog with an IV sticking out of his back. With a serious face, she explained to me how she had "treated" the patient just like I treat her. And that sweet dog had let her. He was a little gray around the nose and a calm dog; I don't think I ever heard him bark. I imagine the removal of the dressing was quite an ordeal for that sweet little guy.

Once this little girl started responding well to the chemo, I discharged her to her family. Her mother was able to take over all her line care and even learned how to perform the blood draws. I hope she recovered well.

The next young patient I had was a pretty twelve-year-old girl who suddenly developed a cancerous tumor in her humerus. Her family was terrified that her identical twin sister might also have the disease, but she was checked and luckily was clear.

The tumor was removed, followed by radiation and chemotherapy. Once again, my job involved line care, performing blood draws, and instructing her mother on sterile dressing changes and blood draws. The patient lost all her hair from the chemo, but adjusted very well. I brought her some wig catalogues, but she preferred wearing different colored scarves and hats.

At first her mom was overwhelmed by all the care her daughter required, but she quickly gained in confidence and competence. A few years after I discharged my patient, her mother called me to report on her daughter and to tell me that she had been so inspired by the services of our agency and the kindness of the nurses that she decided to go back to school to pursue a nursing degree herself. She wanted to help other families as I had helped hers. How nice it was of her to let me know how well her daughter was doing and, most of all, to tell me how much our services had meant to her, inspiring her to change her life!

I received a referral on L, a sweet eleven-year-old girl who had a new colostomy. She had been suffering from Crohn's disease for at least three years, and the uncontrollable diarrhea had damaged the lining of her small intestine. Fortunately, the colostomy was going to be temporary and could be reversed after she healed. My job was to teach her ostomy and diet management. I cannot imagine being eleven and having to deal with such a body image–changing condition. Puberty itself is difficult enough without a colostomy.

When I met L, she was with her mom and seemed very shy. So many doctors, nurses, and specialists at the hospital had been looking at her for the past week, and I could understand her reluctance. I quickly sensed she didn't want someone new examining her. We talked for a while, and I then explained the equipment that she needed to familiarize herself with. But then I noticed her mom. She was totally disengaged in the entire conversation and, over the course of my caring for her daughter, was noticeably absent at most of my follow-up visits. When I finally asked why, my patient told me that her mom had many vague appointments or salon visits for a hair blowout. She was just busy. In retrospect, I believe various clues pointed to her mom having been a high-class call girl.

On one particular visit, her grandmother was there. L had developed a rash on her buttocks and I needed to see it, but she was not about to let me. I tried all kinds of verbal persuasion, to no avail. Finally, her sixty-something-year-old grandmother cut a deal with her. She said, "If I show the nurse my buttocks, will you do the same?" L agreed and her grandmother dropped her drawers. To my amazement, Grandma had on black thong underwear! I did not expect that! I tried to hide my surprise . . . well, at least I hope I did! To be honest, Grandma had pretty good-looking buttocks for her age. That did the trick—L kept her part of the bargain, and I was able to observe her rash and take care of the problem.

This case was difficult for me because L's mom was not your usual concerned parent, and L had so much to deal with. I really felt for her. That type of surgery is life-changing for anyone, and to be faced with it at eleven is really a tough deal. To my amazement, L quickly learned how to manage her appliance, and once her school nurse was updated regarding ostomy management, she returned to school.

She was a very smart and pretty girl, and I hope she did well.

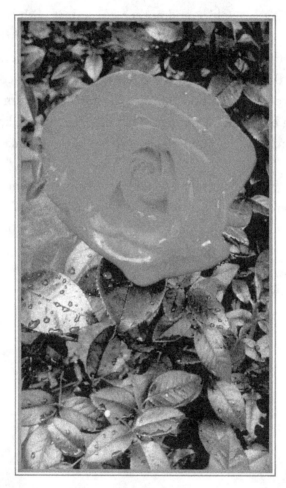

A LASTING LOVE ROSE FROM MY GARDEN.

EIGHT

DEATH

Death comes to us all, but life goes on.

DEATH IS A part of the human condition that we don't seem to talk about much. When I was still in college, I had the opportunity to attend a lecture at Cornell University by Elisabeth Kübler-Ross, a psychiatrist who had recently published her groundbreaking book, *On Death and Dying*, in which she discusses the five stages of grief experienced both by terminal patients and by those left behind to grieve after their death.

My first personal encounter with death occurred when I was eight. My father was killed when his private plane crashed. One day he was there, tucking me into bed at night, and the next day he was gone. As a child, my concerns were vastly different from those of an adult. I worried about who would take me to the father-daughter Girl Scout banquet and what I would do in school when we made Father's Day presents. Thankfully, I had a loving family and dear friends who helped my family through that difficult process of grieving over our loss and the changes to our lives.

When I became a nurse and took care of the terminally ill, I could empathize with families that were facing not only the loss of a loved one, but also all the changes that would occur after the death.

My first encounters with death as a nurse took place during my days and nights working at the hospital when I was still in college. Each situation was unique, and some tested my ability to cope.

When I worked the night shift, I wouldn't put the lights on when I made my rounds. I could shine my flashlight on my white uniform and get enough reflections to see how the patient was doing. Hopefully, they were sleeping. I usually walked through the ward every hour and checked on all my patients. On one particular night, when I did my rounds at 2:00 a.m., everything was fine. At 3:00 a.m., I again checked. However, this time I found a patient sitting bolt upright, staring at me, clearly dead. Startled, I backed out of the room, got a grip, and went back in. Although she obviously had died of natural causes, the sight of her sitting ramrod straight and staring at me gave me quite a jolt. My nurse's aide and I did the aftercare, called the doctor and family, and sent the patient to the morgue. As rattled as I had been, I had forgotten to "toe-tag" her and had to send my nurse's aide down to the morgue to hunt up the body and rectify that oversight.

Another incident occurred in the middle of Christmas Day, when the hospital was teeming with visitors. A beautiful elderly lady had gently passed away, and after her family left, we needed to get her to the morgue. The idea of rolling a sheet-covered patient down the hall through the throngs of visitors gave us pause; I was afraid that we would draw too much attention. This woman looked as though she was peacefully resting, so we fixed her hair, tucked in the sheet around her with her face exposed, placed a pillow beneath her head, and covered her with a nice blanket up to the neck. We successfully got her to the morgue without calling undue attention to the situation.

In all my years as a public health nurse, I only found one person dead at home. She was also a personal friend.

I had been to her home on a Friday and she was doing fine, recovering from a blood clot in her leg. I was doing blood draws twice a week to monitor her anticoagulant therapy. When I pulled into her driveway the following Monday as scheduled, I found the county sheriff already there. Apparently, a neighbor had called because she hadn't seen the normal morning activity at the home.

I walked in, and there sat my sweet patient in her favorite chair, a tissue in her hand, clearly deceased. I called the doctor to report this, along with the estimated time of death. Given the state of her health, we suspected she had died of pulmonary embolism, a blood clot in the lung.

Her sister and brother-in-law, who lived nearby and were at the home, notified the patient's children and then the mortician. As her body was being placed on the gurney to be removed from her home, her sister stopped the activity and asked if we could please pray. The mortician, sheriff, her sister, her brother-in-law, and I all joined hands and recited the Lord's Prayer. It was a very special, profound moment of respect for a loved one.

When someone dies of natural causes in later years of life, it's understandable. It's always sad, but somehow easier to accept as part of the circle of life. However, when children and young folks succumb to a terminal disease, it's difficult to understand and move on.

I took care of a young boy who, at the age of fifteen, was diagnosed with an osteosarcoma. He was a good soccer player, leading a normal life, when he developed a tumor in his leg. The medical tests revealed that it was cancer and would require chemotherapy and radiation.

I became involved in his care after he returned home following initial surgery with a Triple Lumen Hickman in the right side of his chest, a specific catheter used for blood draws and chemotherapy. I instructed his parents on the general maintenance of the line, how to administer IV fluids if needed, and, of course, on strict cleanliness in performing any aspects of his care.

He was a really nice young man, angry at first over this life-threatening disease, but so appreciative of the family and friends who rallied around him. The Make-A-Wish Foundation gave box seats to him, his family, and his friends at a Buffalo Bills game, after which the team came up to meet him and sign autographs. He showed me all the souvenirs and pictures—he was so proud. He also showed me the expensive sneakers he bought to wear with his suit for the junior prom.

For a while, it looked like he might triumph over the disease, but the cancer returned and he was sent to St. Jude for a final attempt to save his life. The attempt failed. This is the hard part for me. To be so closely involved with a family who lost, in this case, their only son. He's gone. And I close the file. His mother called me a few weeks later, wanting to donate unopened supplies that they still had. I quickly went over to remove these unhappy reminders, and we sat and talked about her son. This was a gift to me, an opportunity to have some closure that I wouldn't have gotten otherwise. A young person leaves behind a lasting memory and an overwhelming sadness for a life that ended too soon.

I always felt fortunate that I lived close to my mother and grandparents and was able to care for them right up until they passed.

My grandfather, who really became a surrogate dad to me after my father's passing, was diagnosed with terminal colon cancer. My grandmother wanted to bring him home, which is also what he wanted. So with the assistance of hospice, that's what we did. I was able to be with him right until the end.

We had had a big snowstorm that March and I wasn't able to get down to their home for a few days. On Sunday, I asked my husband, "Will you drive me down there?" When I got there, I gave Gramps a good bath, changed his bed, and was gratified to see him looking great. My husband, Jim, went in to see him, they had a nice conversation, and we left. Later that evening, my grandmother called to tell me that he wasn't doing too well, so I went back. He was semicomatose and restless. I kept turning him over, trying to make him comfortable. I did this for about five hours and told Grandma, "He's dying." She understood. At about 11:30, he finally settled, and I asked Grandma if she'd like me to spend the night. She said, "No, go home. I'll be all right." I did . . . reluctantly.

I was in bed, finally able to sleep after some tossing and turning. At 2:00 a.m., I awoke with a start. Then the phone rang. I knew what the news was before I picked up. Gramps had died. I called my sister and went back over to Grandma's, where my sister met me. Grandpa was positioned quietly on his side. My sister, who is a teacher, said, "Can I see him? I've never seen a dead person before." The three of us—my sister, Grandma, and I—stood around his bed looking at the peaceful figure before us. My sister said, "Are you sure he's dead?" Well, my no-nonsense grandmother slapped his face and said, "Of course, he's dead. Deader than a stone!" We were shocked, to say the least. Here is the love of her life, the man she's been married to for more than fifty years, and yet she immediately grasps and accepts the reality of his death.

My grandmother lived for another fifteen years, until the age of 103. She was really something, living home alone until she was 98, then living her final years in a skilled nursing facility. I'd have tea with her one or two times a week, and every time, she'd tell the ladies at her table, "This is my granddaughter, and she's a nurse!" They'd all respond, "We know, Grace. You already told us that!" Over time, she just faded away—quietly, ready to die. I think of my grandparents often and I still miss them every day.

My mother, on the other hand, was a different story. I half expected her to live as long as her mother, as she really had no health issues. But she smoked. All my life I tried to get her to quit, but she could not and would not. One afternoon, she called me from the doctor's office. She had a cold, went to her doctor, and had a chest X-ray. He found a tumor in her lung. That was not something she was prepared to hear. I met her at his office and we talked, and she agreed to see a specialist.

Although concerned about side effects, my mother agreed to try chemotherapy, with the proviso that if she wanted to stop at any time, she could. She underwent the treatment for about six months, then one day after her visit to the lab, she turned to me and said, "That's all. I want hospice. I'm done."

By that time we had hired round-the-clock help in her home. Hospice nurses began to come in as well. I had retired by that point but was still working part-time as a contract nurse, and I could go every evening to make her supper and supervise her meds. One morning, the hospice nurse called me at work and said that my mom was not doing well, and I'd better come to see her. I left work and found Mom coherent but with labored breathing. I called my sister and was glad that we could all be there together. During those difficult hours, Mom would get restless, but we were able to reposition her to make her more comfortable. The hospice nurse had also started morphine, which greatly helped.

When the pain intensified, Mom would ask for more medication. At first, I'd check my notebook to make sure it wasn't too soon. Then it dawned on me, "So what? She's dying. Let her be comfortable." It's hard to be objective when the patient is a loved one, and especially hard when that loved one is your mother.

Mom was finally positioned well and breathing quietly. She could no longer move herself. The private caregiver and I were sitting near her bed when suddenly my mother sat up and reached for the sky, as though someone was coming down to get her. Then she lay back in the bed—dead. I was astonished. I couldn't believe it. I took my stethoscope, placed it on her chest, and confirmed that she was indeed gone. I comfort myself with the thought that, after all those years, my dad had come down to get her, and they were finally together again.

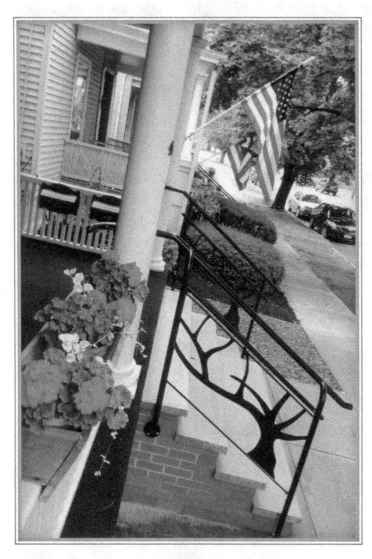

A PICTURE OF MY PORCH STEPS AND STREET.

NINE

HOMES REFLECT THEIR OWNERS

Listen and observe. Be a bit curious about the people you treat,
and you may be amazed by what is revealed.

OFTEN WHEN I told acquaintances that I was a home health nurse, the first thing they'd say is, "I bet you go into some terrible places." And I did.

A few patients, for example, were hoarders. They needed things around them and could not part with anything, not even a newspaper. It's difficult working with a patient under these circumstances, but I did the best I could and made sure I informed the doctor so that he or she would know what limitations I faced in the home. It was only when the hoarding presented a true health and safety hazard that I'd call Adult Protective Services or the local fire department to intervene.

While it's true that some home situations were less than ideal, I also saw some of the most beautiful homes in the county, which inspired me in my own home decoration. The artistic choices people made for display in their homes often led to interesting revelations about their pasts and created stronger bonds between us.

I once read that one of our greatest, underappreciated natural resources is our elderly. I always kept that in my mind. I loved hearing people's stories and enjoyed drawing my patients out with a few questions: How did you meet your wife? What was your occupation? How long have you lived on this farm? The inspiration for many of my questions often came from looking around their homes. I've only given a few examples here, but I believe that every person, every life, has a story—maybe more than one!

When I go into people's homes, I notice their decor and their collections. People display their treasures. After introducing myself, getting paperwork and charting started, performing a complete physical assessment, and providing the needed care, I would engage in a bit of conversation with the patient, oftentimes referencing what I saw around me in the home.

In one home, a huge pair of wooden skis was displayed on the living room wall. I had to ask. It turns out that the patient had been an elite member of the WWII ski patrol in Europe. He told me how he learned to ski out west in America and then was sent over to the Alps to fight the Germans. The patrol wore all-white uniforms as a form of camouflage and skied with their rifles and gear on their backs. How fascinating!

Another time I walked into a lovely apartment and saw hanging on the wall a flag from the Augusta National Golf Club in Georgia. I'm a golfer, so I understood the rarity of someone in our town having a flag from the Masters. He not only had the flag, but the wooden pole as well. He had acquired the flag after twenty years of attending the Masters, and a groundskeeper he befriended obtained it for him.

Several mechanical engineer patients impressed me over the years with the modifications they made to their homes. One gentleman rewired his home so that he could control the lights for each room from just one switch, long before "smart homes" and Alexa. Another guy had an old farmhouse with an unusual bathroom situation. Apparently, the previous owner had converted a small bedroom into a large bathroom, but there were three doors to the room. The patient devised a locking system so one could close the door and lock all three doors from any one of the doors. So clever!

So many of my clients had beige, neutral living rooms, drapes, and carpets. Other clients had an ability to use color and mix prints. I found their homes cheerful and welcoming and was inspired to make similar changes in my home.

I received a referral on MB, a lovely lady who lived about forty miles from the main office. I pulled up to this cute white bungalow that even had a white picket fence around the yard. Since I was driving my blue Caddy at the time, her husband came right out to meet me. We exchanged greetings, and then I stepped inside. What a sight! I never saw such a cute house in my life.

After the initial exam and paperwork had been completed, I asked MB if she had hired a professional interior decorator. She said, "No. All the curtains, pillows, and accent quilts I made myself." Her sense of color was phenomenal. The way she combined different flowered fabrics with striped wallpaper was enchanting. What an artistic eye she had! That warm, beautiful home made quite an impression on me. I made the decision then and there that when decorating my own home, I would not shy away from vibrant colors. I have hues of red, pink, blue, and green throughout my home thanks to the inspiration of MB.

M, a patient I followed for many years who had uncontrollable hypertension, also had an impressive sense of color. She lived in a small Cape

Cod–style home, tastefully filled with antiques. In her living room, she somehow managed gold and white wallpaper, orange carpet, red oriental rugs, pink drapes, and a cranberry couch and chair to stunning effect. All these colors combined just worked! Going up the stairs was black carpeting with red and pink roses—just beautiful. She, too, did all her own decorating, but as she was not a seamstress, she had her drapes and pillows made. I just loved going to visit her in that comfortable, striking living room. Today, I have a front entrance inspired by M. The walls are a dark red with white trim, and going up the stairs is a navy carpet with red and pink roses.

I have great gratitude for these two women, MB and M. When I look around my home, I think of them and smile. Without their inspiring, bold decorating choices, I don't think I would have had the courage to use so much color in my own home. How boring life would have been without it!

One of the most beautiful homes I visited belonged to L, a retired attorney who was a widow. She was not able to ambulate on her own due to latent polio, so she used a scooter outside and inside to get around. Because her large Victorian home had an elevator, she was able to access all the parts of her home. I met L when her doctor ordered daily cleansing, packing, and dressing changes to her hip because of an infection deep in the joint. This care continued for about two years, and we became good friends.

Although L had a cleaning lady and an occasional cook, L's children were concerned about her living on her own in that big house. They arranged for a male nursing student from the local hospital to board in her home at night. L was not too pleased with this situation and had concerns about her new boarder. One day, she asked me if I could check every room in her home and let her know if everything was okay. I did as she asked and discovered in the back bedroom, where he was staying, a mess of chip bags, pop cans, and take-out containers. Clearly, he was not a respectful tenant. I reported back to my client, who asked him to leave later that day.

The next day, she had her cleaning lady clean up the mess and informed her children that "she was just fine on her own." Once she reclaimed her home, she called and invited me over to have a gin and tonic with her. I went, of course, and she confided that she had a G&T every day at one in the afternoon, just like the Queen Mum! Even after she was no longer my patient, we remained friends, and I stayed in contact with her until she died.

One other home display that stands out to me was a curio cabinet in the home of a retired gaffer (glassblower), the husband of my patient. As a result of his years working with glass, he had multiple scars on his forearms where hot glass and sparks had hit above his gloves. That lighted curio cabinet, with a mirrored back, just sparkled in their living room and was filled with the most beautiful glass objects. They were all original designs of his that did not make the cut for mass production—and had survived the company's policy of smashing any design that wasn't accepted. He loved being a gaffer and couldn't bring himself to destroy the pieces he had created.

He once removed one of his precious designs from the cabinet and showed it to me. It was a gorgeous, clear glass Civil War cannon, approximately ten inches long by five inches wide. It was absolutely beautiful! He had designed it to commemorate the 1976 bicentennial. Unfortunately, it hadn't made the cut because the piece was too costly and time consuming to make. All of his pieces were magnificent works of art!

I asked one time what he thought all that glass would be worth now. He had no idea, but suspected it would be "a lot." He willed all of it to his children. What a treasure they inherited!

One springtime in the seventies, I received a new referral on an elderly woman who required monthly B12 injections. When I finally found her home, I realized it was newly built and was at the end of a cul-de-sac. The home was gorgeous. It was all on one floor, with a sloping roofline and a monstrous wooden front door. When I knocked, a tall, middle-aged blonde woman greeted me with a beautiful German accent and escorted me inside. I'll refer to her as G, and from that first meeting, she always called me Miss Linda. She was lovely!

Her mother was the patient. When G escorted me into her mother's bedroom, quite a picture was before me. I had never seen such massive and spectacular wooden bedroom furniture in my life. Propped up in the middle of the large bed was an eighty-something, silver-haired woman wearing a white lace nightgown under a lavender crocheted bed jacket. A silver tray with the remnants of her breakfast was sitting on the bed next to her. Since she did not speak a word of English, her daughter introduced me to her in German and explained that I would be visiting her monthly to give her a much needed injection. I followed this lovely lady for almost two years.

Sometimes after my visit the ladies would give me German chocolate candy bars, which were divine. I'd eat them in the car as I headed to my next visit. I couldn't help myself!

That Christmas season, they invited my mother and me to their house after work for a drink and to help them decorate their Christmas tree. What a wonderful evening we had. While Mom and I enjoyed Canadian Club with water on the rocks served in gorgeous crystal glasses along with exquisite holiday cookies, we helped them place the most beautiful Christmas ornaments on their tree. It was just an ideal Christmas celebration. As a gift that year, the ladies gave me my first bottle of Chanel No. 5.

As you can probably tell, I truly enjoyed my visits there. One time, I arrived right after we had had a big snowstorm. About two feet of fresh white snow was all around, and when I approached the front door, I noticed all of the oriental carpets from the front hall were lying in the snow. When G answered the door, I asked, "Why are the carpets in the snow?" She told me that the reflection of the sun on the new snow brightens the colors in the carpets. It was something they always did back in Germany.

When I learned that I was being transferred and that another nurse was taking my place, I said a sad goodbye to these ladies. We had coffee, my first espresso (which I did not like but drank anyway to be polite), and, with a tearful goodbye, parted. I kept tabs on them through the agency. G stayed in the house after her mother passed and became active in her community library.

We are blessed in this area to have many beautiful lakes. My usual nursing assignments were never at the lakes full-time, but every now and then I would get a referral, usually when I was on-call, to make a visit to one of them.

D was recovering from triple bypass surgery and was staying with his daughter, who had a beautiful home right on the lake. When I called for directions, she told me to pull in the driveway, park, and then enter through the garage. The house sat on the water, right in front of this massive garage. As I was walking through it, I noticed all of these interesting tools—drill presses, vices, sanders, metal shafts, and grips—and guessed it was equipment to make golf clubs.

Then I walked into the house and saw the lake through the windows. The view stretched all across the front of the house—it went on forever. I was mesmerized. What a treat it would be just to stand in the kitchen and do the dishes while enjoying the view!

After meeting the patient and performing my nursing assessment, I had to ask about the garage. D started talking and confirmed that he and his son-in-law did indeed make personalized golf clubs. As the conversation continued, his daughter said that she recognized my name and that she had been in high school with my husband when he was enrolled in their school for a short time. She still remembered him, so that says a lot for him! I think I spent almost two hours with them on that Saturday, just visiting.

My next visit was a different story. D's daughter called to say that he had developed the strangest problem. I quickly drove out there for a follow-up visit. When I saw the problem, I knew exactly what she meant. Two very large blisters had formed on the tops of both of his feet, covering the entire dorsal surface. I had never seen anything like it before. I told them not to break the blisters and that I'd call the doctor to see what was going on.

Apparently, D needed to expel more fluid from his body than his kidneys could manage, so the fluid came out of the skin in the form of those large blisters. We treated them daily for several weeks with Silvadene cream and dry sterile dressings until they finally deflated and he could wear regular slippers again. Those blisters turned out to be more of an issue than his bypass surgery.

D stayed with his daughter for quite some time, as normally he lived alone in a trailer. It was always a real pleasure visiting him on the lake. That view out of the front picture window was breathtaking and so relaxing. I believe water can truly change one's mood.

During my visits to D, I not only got to see a panoramic view of the lake and learn some amusing high school gossip about my husband, but

I also gained some more fascinating knowledge about the human body. It is a marvelous machine that tries to rectify and heal itself as much as possible.

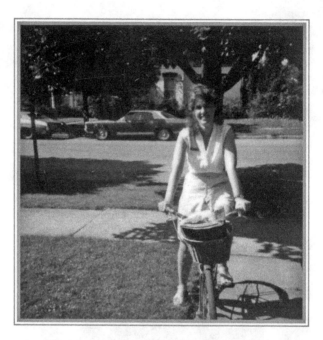

ME ON MY BICYCLE, MAKING HOME VISITS.

TEN

CHANGES IN PUBLIC HEALTH NURSING
OVER THE YEARS

Change is inevitable. Find a way to adapt to new rules and regulations, while still keeping the goal in mind: helping the patient.

WHEN I FIRST went to work for the county nursing service, nurses were assigned a geographic work area within the county borders. Any referrals from doctors, hospitals, or the community for that geographic area were covered by the assigned nurse. If the area became too busy, other nearby nurses would assist.

We were all reimbursed for our mileage. Once you were in your area, driving time was usually minimal, except for in the outlying country areas, where driving time between patients could be thirty to forty minutes. My first fifteen to twenty years were spent in the city, so driving long distances was not an issue. In fact, one summer I was given permission through the risk management office to ride my bike when the visits were not complicated and I wouldn't need my medical bag. Usually I could ride my bike at least three times a week. The patients really got a kick out of seeing me pull up to their homes on my bike with a notepad, stethoscope, and blood pressure cuff all in my basket.

At one time, I believe we had eleven nurses just in the small city alone, and we would each carry a caseload of twenty to forty patients. That changed immensely over the years. As the Medicare rules and regulations required more detailed documentation for reimbursement, more time was needed on paperwork. And as hospital stays became shorter, sending patients home sicker, the patient population grew. As an example, in 1977, open-heart surgery was in its infancy, and a usual hospital stay was four to six weeks. In the eighties, this surgery was now routine, and patients often returned home just three days after surgery.

Though there were changes as the number and nature of patients changed over the years, our focus always was keeping patients safe and healthy in their own homes as long as possible. With more acutely ill people coming home sooner, we changed to an acute care agency. In other words, our patient population changed from mainly elderly patients, requiring palliative or long-term care, to patients of all ages with diverse medical needs. These patients tended to need the services of a public health nurse for a shorter length of time, usually no more than three to four weeks.

The improvements that were made in technology and diagnostics increased the outpatient business in most hospitals. This meant we were receiving referrals on patients with more acute needs. By the end of my career, I was seeing and treating patients in their own homes who would have been in the intensive care unit thirty years ago.

Back in 1975, a cholecystectomy (gallbladder removal) patient would routinely spend two weeks in intensive care following surgery and then another one to two weeks in the hospital on a standard surgical floor. By the time he returned home, his incisions would be completely healed. Currently, a cholecystectomy is an outpatient procedure or a one- to two-day stay in the hospital. It's done laparoscopically, and the patient goes home with only two to three minor incisions, which are covered with Band-Aids.

In the early eighties, AIDS was a serious problem. Due to the contagious nature of the disease and its personal ramifications, strict confidentiality was required. Because the protection of patient privacy was deemed paramount, it was possible that a caregiver might be unaware that a patient had infectious HIV. Consequently, all patients had to be treated, regardless of their known and unknown diagnoses, as though each had infectious HIV. This caused a major change in how medical personnel dealt with patients.

When I started as a public health nurse, I would wash my hands before drawing blood or giving injections. Now gloves were required before every procedure that had the potential of contact with bodily fluids. Our home health aides had to wear gloves to give bed baths and apply lotion. It was truly an adjustment to function with gloves on.

I found this change to be rather sad. There is something therapeutic in the touch of another human being. Sometimes public health nurses and home health aides were the only human touch our patients had. The gloves put up a barrier between the nurse and patient that weakened that interaction. It is understandable that universal precautions be taught and taken when faced with the possible spread of a contagion, be it AIDS, scabies, lice, TB, or other disease. And I certainly did not want to risk carrying a disease home to my family. However, I felt that my patients craved that human touch, and when their care was done and no bodily fluids were present, I frequently removed my gloves and placed a hand on them or hugged them.

Changes in Medicare, or in the interpretations of Medicare, over the years also resulted in many of the changes in home health care. Medicare was started in 1965, mainly as a way of assisting the elderly with health care costs. When I started in the seventies, home health care under Medicare was expanding as patients with chronic illnesses, not necessarily elderly, were now eligible under Medicare. Home health care was viewed at this time as (1) more humane, allowing patients to be in the comfort of their homes; (2) able to provide care for conditions that did not require hospitalization; and (3) more cost effective than hospitals. In the eighties, benefits were further expanded, but other issues created more problems, causing many claims to be denied. This led to a lawsuit, which resulted in some changes and clarification in wording. In the nineties, higher health care costs brought about other changes and cuts in Medicare and home health care funding based on "arbitrary criteria" and "agency cost history." At this time, concerns arose about consistency and fraudulent practices. In the 2000s, a new system was introduced, one that changed how payments were calculated, relying heavily on new "Outcomes and Assessment" documentation. What all of this meant for me was more paperwork, more time at my desk, more hoops to jump through, and more regulations about what I could and could not do for patients.

The demand for more detailed information due to all of these fast-paced changes in medical procedures and in Medicare requirements and oversight meant that a laptop computer became an absolute necessity. That was another adjustment I had to make. I was so used to having conversation with each individual patient, all the while observing each for changes or improvements and the like. I was not comfortable staring at a computer screen as I recorded answers to my questions. I found a way to document some things on the computer, interact with the patient, and then fill in the blanks as I sat in my car after the visit. I just didn't want to lose that personal connection with my patients. I refused to accept that it was inevitable that technology would separate me from my patients.

When I first started, we had patients we followed for twenty or more years. We interacted more with our patients and created a bond. In later years, we followed patients in three- to four-week intervals.

The working principle today is "the sooner they get better, the faster the discharge, the better it is for the agency." In theory, this is fine. But in practice, things aren't always that straightforward.

For example, after a knee replacement, hip surgery, bypass surgery, or cholecystectomy, patients in the forty- to seventy-year-old range can and do heal quickly. But for those patients in their upper eighties and older, recuperation takes much longer. Most folks in this age bracket also have other chronic conditions such as arthritis, diabetes, vision and hearing problems, COPD, and possibly obesity.

I enjoyed the challenge of trying to get patients as healthy as possible through assessments, health education, lifestyle changes, and medication monitoring. Of course, there were normal hospital discharges—wound healing and other issues when patients first come home—but teaching them and their caregivers to live the best life they can while managing their chronic illness was really my goal. Some folks did very well. Others, not so much. When I would discharge the "not so much" patients, I knew I'd see them again soon, but the regulations and protocols required their discharge from our services.

In addition to the changes in paperwork, computer use, and Medicare reimbursement, there also were huge advances in medical technology. The most remarkable one that I encountered involved caring for a patient who was on the heart transplant list and had an external heart pump in place. Our job was to draw his blood weekly and assess for any signs of possible infection at the pump insertion site.

It is surreal placing a stethoscope on a living, breathing patient with an external heart in place. There is no pulse. Yet, here is the patient, up and about, talking to you, and all you can hear in your stethoscope is a whirring sound in his chest. No heartbeat! After I retired, I lost track of the patient and don't know if he ever received the new heart. It is amazing to think of how far science and technology have advanced over the years. I wonder what new medical marvels are in store for us.

Although I adapted to the changes in patient load, patient type, stricter procedures to prevent spreading disease, changes in Medicare, and much more paperwork, I tried to maintain a personal connection of some kind with the patient, because that is often as important as the medical care itself. I am sure as the years pass more and more changes in medicine will continue to make the job even more fascinating than it is today. Never a dull moment!

ELEVEN
SPECIAL CASES

As much as you give, you also receive—in gratitude,
appreciation, and friendship.

I WAS FORTUNATE to start my job at a time when I had more free-dom to interact with my patients. So many of the folks I met over the years touched my heart and made lasting impressions. I remember with fondness some of the funny, strange, or sweet moments that I had with a few of these individuals.

Sweet E was ninety-four and had just been released from the hospital. If I recall correctly, she had a fractured hip. This was my one and only visit to her. She was new to a walker and needed home physical therapy. At that time, the public health nurses always did the initial evaluation, and then physical therapy took over the case. E was a very spry elderly lady. She stood less than five feet tall and could fit right under my arm. As I was interviewing her, I asked about the sign out front of her home

THESE PATIENTS ARE FOREVER IN MY HEART.

that read "Erma's." She had a stand out in front of her family's grape-vines where she sold grape pies. I marveled that she was still baking at her age. She planned to get back at it as soon as her hip was healed. E proceeded to tell me that baking her grape pies was easy, and she loved doing it. She then gave me a printed recipe. That's when I had to confess, "I have never baked a pie." Sweet E reached over, slapped my leg, and said, "Well, you're gonna need help!" I laughed so hard I almost dropped my laptop. Needless to say, I never did bake a grape pie!

EN was an eighty-year-old widower who lived in a little bungalow behind his niece's home. After his wife passed away, he had built the little three-room house behind what was then his sister's home. His sister and her family watched out for him, but when his sister passed away, his niece took over the job. The niece was the one who made the referral to public health nursing. She had noticed that EN had become more reclusive, refusing to attend family get-togethers, and he had not seen a doctor in many years. The family also noticed a foul odor about him and his little house, which made them all the more concerned.

When I attempted my first visit, I had some trouble finding the place. Finally, I walked into the backyard of the address I was given and saw his sweet little bungalow. After knocking, I entered his home, and the first thing I noticed was the terrible odor. Immediately, I tried to ignore the smell, as I did not want to offend EN. It was quickly evident that the odor was coming from his person.

I was somewhat surprised that the home itself was neat and clean. I proceeded into his living room and noticed that the ceilings, which were very low, were painted a bright orange. I instinctively ducked down. Those colored ceilings surprised me, but somehow it seemed to work with his brown paneling. I had to remark on the color, and EN was so proud to tell me he had built and decorated the home himself.

I suggested we walk into the kitchen so I could place my barrier with my nursing bag on the table. Then I could do a complete physical assessment along with the necessary paperwork. EN stood by the table with his checked flannel button-down shirt and too-large green work pants hiked up high above his waist, all cinched together with a black leather belt. I noted a large bulge protruding from the left side of his lower abdomen. After checking his vital signs and lung sounds, I asked if I could see his colostomy. EN had told me he had had that bowel surgery about fifteen years ago. He loosened his pants and dropped his trousers, and what I saw was unbelievable.

EN had a prolapsed colostomy with about one and a half feet of small intestine on the outside of his body. He had it all collected up in a small white garbage bag, held together with an old-style ostomy ring and belt. Actually, it was quite ingenious, as his old appliance bags were way too small to hold that much intestine. The origin of the odor was obvious. I needed to correct this ASAP!

Colostomy management and equipment had come a long way in the last ten years. The latest barrier products with odor management and new skin-friendly adhesives made colostomy care much easier and more comfortable for the patient. But the first thing EN needed was to see a surgeon and have his prolapsed bowel corrected.

At my next visit, I brought with me the latest in ostomy equipment so he could see exactly what I was talking about. I then demonstrated how to use the bags and flanges. I left all the supplies there so he could familiarize himself with them. This was going to be a big change for him.

I was soon successful in convincing him to see a local surgeon. After surgery, he had a normal stomach. His abdomen was flat, with a small rosette stoma on the lower left side. I performed his ostomy care for a short while and eventually taught him to be independent with his bag changes, but the flange management twice a week was too difficult for him. I visited him every Tuesday and Friday for many years, and in that time, we had a lot of great conversations. He especially enjoyed my visits at Christmastime, when I would bring my mom and give him some homemade banana bread. I think I still have the tawny port he gave me for Christmas one year. He told me that was the last bottle of booze he bought before quitting drinking many years ago.

Because he lived alone, EN was unaware of the advances that had been made in medical appliances. Those improvements made a huge change in his life. He was a sweet little guy who became a dear friend.

EW was a dear gentleman who was a retired machinist from the Erie Railroad. He was also quite the history buff.

EW was extremely hard-of-hearing. I believe the original referral on him came from his neighbors, who were concerned that he wasn't eating well, was quite feeble, and might not be safe alone. When I went to visit him for the first time, I could understand their concerns. On his door were signs proclaiming: "I AM VERY DEAF" and "JUST WALK IN." It was like he was asking to be robbed.

I did an assessment. At that time, in the late seventies and early eighties, I was able to admit patients to our services for just routine checks—vitals and the like—and home health aide services to help with bathing and activities of daily living. He flourished once he got the assistance he needed.

I visited him every two weeks, per state law, for many years. In that time, we became friends. Through our conversations, I discovered that he was an Academy graduate, and so was I. Knowing that, I asked EW and his doctor if he could attend The Academy alumni banquet dinner that May as my date. I was twenty-four and he was eighty-four. The answer was yes from both the patient and doctor. What a hoot! When I came to pick him up, EW was dressed in his best brown suit, which was a little too big, a starched white shirt, and a brown-and-gold striped tie. He looked so dapper. When we arrived at the banquet, the alumni president made special seating arrangements for us, placing us closer to the food so that EW wouldn't have to walk too far to the buffet. EW had the time of his life. He thanked me for that evening every time I visited until he died.

He gave me two very special Christmas gifts in the years following. One was a pair of earrings he had made for his wife, fashioned out of Mercury head dimes. I had them changed into pierced earrings so I could wear them. The other was a periodical documenting the flood of '72, with all the corrections he had made in it. He was a fussy little guy, but always right!

Nowadays, a public health nurse couldn't do what I did for him; it would not be allowed. A rather sad change in caring for a patient.

G was the dearest little octogenarian, with bad arthritis and mild deafness and hypertension. She was a widow with no children, living in the cutest little crooked house. The porch slanted, the kitchen tilted, but the home was clean as a whistle.

G needed cataract surgery at a time when the procedure required an overnight stay in the hospital. Post-op treatment consisted of eye drops in the morning, sunglasses as needed, and eye ointment and a bandage at night. Because the eye dressing can cause blurry vision and depth perception to be off, the drops and ointment were difficult for a patient to administer by herself. For two weeks, G was my first patient in the morning, when she would get eye drops, and my last patient on my way home, when she would get the ointment and eye bandage. Once her eye healed, she was so thrilled that she could see the bright, vivid colors of her flower garden. She remarked to me, "Now I can see your blue eyes."

G wasn't a churchgoer, as getting out was difficult for her. But she was religious, and she regularly watched Oral Roberts on TV. One day she got a letter from Oral Roberts University asking for money. G was a very frugal person, living and managing her household on just Social Security. Her only extravagance was in spoiling her fat tiger cat. As tight as money was, she still managed to save a little (but did not donate anything to Oral Roberts). When I arrived at her home one day for my scheduled visit, I found her fuming and sputtering over the fact that Oral Roberts was asking her for money for his wife's cataract surgery. G proclaimed, "I just had that done and nobody gave me any extra money." This independent, hardworking woman was shocked at the notion that the Roberts family expected others to do for them what she was able to do for herself.

Easter was approaching, and I asked G if she would like to go to church with my mother and me, followed by dinner at Mom's. She accepted. When I picked her up, I found her all decked out in the nicest cotton dress, polished white shoes, and a navy coat. I think it was the first time I'd seen her without an apron on. We arrived at the church and got seated in Mom's usual pew. The service had just started, and in order for G to better hear the minister's opening prayer, she turned her hearing aids way up. When the first hymn began, we all stood up, and my mother's beautiful but very loud voice came booming out. Well, G grabbed her ears fast and quickly turned those hearing aids down. I smiled through the whole service. It was such a treat being there for Easter with two lovely ladies, and the enjoyment of their company continued through dinner. This is another instance that today's restrictions wouldn't allow.

That fall, I had some minor surgery and was off work for about two weeks. G saw my name in the paper and wanted to send a get-well card. Being her frugal self, she used what she had on hand. I received a Disneyland postcard with a get-well wish written on the back. How cute is that! She sweetly expressed how much she missed me and that she hoped I was doing well. I've kept the card and read it again just the other day. Dear G lived to her mid-nineties and died quietly at home. She always has a place in my heart.

MT was an extremely well-educated lady who ended up in one of the county's small towns when she married. When I met her, she was a widow with no children and no relatives nearby. As she aged, she had become increasingly hard of hearing, which in turn made her more reclusive. She had pernicious anemia and required a monthly vitamin B12 injection, which is why I became involved with her care. Because of her hearing loss, she was afraid and kept her doors locked. This made her difficult to visit: She sometimes couldn't hear me knocking at her door.

One day, a nursing student and I went to visit MT. Fortunately, we didn't have a difficult time getting her to answer the door. We had our usual chat, which she could follow as long as she was looking at me. I then went to the kitchen to get the vial of B12 out of the refrigerator. I opened the door, and *boom!*—a mouse dropped to the floor at my feet and scurried away. Startled, I jumped back pretty fast. The student nurse, eyes wide in panic, half jumped out of her chair. I figured the mouse was sitting in the egg tray, and when I opened the door, he lost his balance and fell out. I had to find out how that mouse got in that refrigerator. I took a good look inside and discovered that the drain cover in the bottom of the refrigerator was missing, allowing that mouse to crawl in, eat my patient's Meals on Wheels, and depart. To correct this problem, I arranged for a home health aide to come to the house the next day, and together we cleaned out and repaired the fridge. Sometimes you have to do a little extra for folks.

The mouse in the fridge was certainly an event to remember, but it turned out not to be the most memorable day in my dealings with MT. One summer day when I went to visit, I smelled gas as I walked up the porch steps, and I found her door open. My eyes burned and watered terribly as I entered the house. MT was sleeping soundly on the sofa and never heard me enter. I checked around, and on the stove in her kitchen was a teakettle, but the burner under it was not lit. The pilot light had gone out, and gas continued to pour into the house. I immediately shut off the stove, woke MT, helped her to the porch, and called the gas company's emergency phone number. I opened as many doors and windows as I could and waited for the gas man.

When he got to the house, he did not seem as concerned as I was, but by then much of the gas had dissipated. He dismantled the stove and left. I explained everything to my patient as best as I could and made a few calls on her behalf, one to a niece who planned to visit her and help her out and one to the stove repairman. MT was a lovely lady, but it was obvious that her living alone was not a good idea anymore. I was very happy that her niece stepped in to help out and made arrangements for her to go into an adult-care facility near her. She needed some supervision, and placement in an assisted-living situation was the right answer.

K was a retired milk hauler. He drove all around the surrounding counties, collecting milk from the local farmers and delivering it to the dairy. Since K loved to chat, I imagine he thoroughly enjoyed standing outside and visiting with the farmers as his truck filled at the milk house. I'm quite sure all of that sun exposure over the years was the probable cause of the skin cancer on his head, face, and nose.

Once these lesions were surgically removed, I started visiting him for the aftercare. The sites on his nose weren't healing, and after follow-up appointments with his plastic surgeon, the doctor regrettably found it necessary to remove his entire nose. That was the first time I had ever seen that. It was so strange to look straight into a face and see just the reddish-pink septum of the nose and two red holes leading into his head. His profile was even stranger with no nose jutting out below the forehead and brow. As I was cleaning his wound one day, it occurred to me that the site was exposed to any number of foreign objects: a piece of lint, a hair, or a fly. When I contacted the doctor about the danger, I was shocked to discover there were no plans to protect the open nose holes. I pondered the situation that night and resolved to make K a nose cover.

When I told K my idea at the next visit, he agreed to work with me. In addition to being a milk hauler, K was also an amateur artist. He took foam trays, the kind found under meat at grocery stores, painted them flat white as a background, then sketched country scenes on them. He then glued magnets to the back so that they could be displayed on refrigerators. I still have the one he gave me.

The nose cover project presented a new artistic challenge for him. We looked around his kitchen and found a plastic tub that had been for butter. We cut the bottom off and placed the plastic in the microwave for one to two minutes to soften it. I then cut a triangle that was slightly elongated with a tab at the top, so I could connect it to the bridge of his glasses. I then bent the piece in half to create a tent-like appearance. Because the yellowish-beige color of the nose cover did not look good against K's skin tone, he decided to cover it with a flesh-colored moleskin, which blended well with his skin's coloring. We taped the tab of the device to the bridge of his glasses, trimmed the bottom of the triangle to fit his face, and voilà, we had a plastic nose to cover his surgical scar. Both K and I were pleased with the result. I was also happy that the device provided safety and cleanliness, and K was thrilled that he could go out in public without getting a multitude of stares.

On my last visit, over coffee, K told me a funny story. Earlier in the week he was at a grocery store and noticed a little girl, about eight, looking at his face. K took off his glasses and yelled, "Boo!" Well, I guess she jumped a mile. He then told her what had happened to him and explained the nose cover. I was gratified that the device had restored some of his self-confidence, allowing him to mingle in public and not retreat from society. I always wondered what his doctor thought about his butter tub moleskin nose when K went back for checkups. It confounded me that a plastic surgeon would remove a nose completely without supplying a prosthesis. Our makeshift device did the trick.

I visited VS every two weeks to supervise her home health aide and to monitor her diabetes. She loved to visit and always had a story to tell.

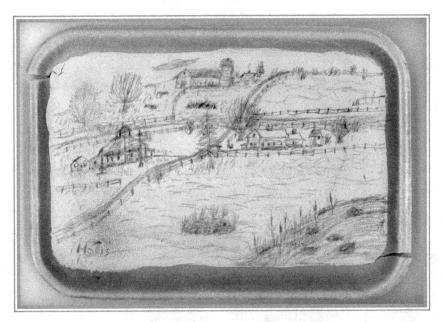

THE STYROFOAM ART K GAVE ME.

About once a month, I'd soak her feet and give her a pedicure while assessing her skin, nails, and the bottoms of her feet. I had been visiting her for about four to five years when I learned she had been admitted to the hospital with a cerebrovascular accident—that is, a stroke. When I went to a discharge planning session, I learned that her stroke was quite extensive and that she was still in the ICU.

After a few weeks passed, the skilled nursing facility where VS was recovering requested that I make a pre-discharge visit at the facility. My knowledge of her condition prior to her hospitalization would help me assess whether it was safe to discharge her back to her home. I was excited to see her, but I had no idea how her condition had changed since her stroke or if she would remember me. When I arrived at the nursing home, I found VS waiting for me. I learned that the stroke had affected her speech, and even though she was receiving speech therapy, she was having difficulty putting sentences together. When I walked into her room, she recognized me immediately. VS beamed and exclaimed, "God bless America!" We both laughed and cried. VS's daughter was there and we talked about her needs. I had VS get out of her chair, walk, go into and out of the bathroom, and get in and out of her bed. Physically, she did very well, but the speech was a problem. She wouldn't be safe at home alone since she would be unable to communicate effectively if she had a problem. VS was dearly loved by her family and friends, and her family developed a plan to rotate supervision of her so that she could come home. She was able to live there several more years thanks to their care.

On Christmas about a year before her stroke, VS had given me a pair of beautiful pillowcases that she had crocheted and embroidered. They were too beautiful to use—I still have them in the original box in a drawer in my guest bedroom. Periodically, I take them out to admire them and think, "God bless America" made these for me.

JG was a lovely man who lived with his wife in a nice home. He had wounds on his lower legs due to poor circulation and required dressing changes two times a day. The skin on his lower legs was almost nonexistent, which made removing the old dressings extremely painful for him. After the dressing removal, I would apply Silvadene ointment, cover with a Vaseline dressing to keep the skin moist, and finally wrap the legs with a Kling gauze dressing.

JG and I figured out that when I first arrived, I would soak his dressings with sterile water, let them sit for about ten to fifteen minutes, and then carefully pull them off before applying the new dressings. It took longer, but was much more comfortable for him. He really seemed to like me, as I tried to be so gentle with him. I knew by the condition of his skin and his apparent poor circulation that those dressing changes were painful. As his care progressed, I eventually taught his wife the procedure so that she could do the second dressing in the evening. Once, while I was taking care of him, JG said, "If there was ever a wife store and you were in it, I'd pick you." He was a charmer!

On one of my visits, I found JG lethargic, with his eyes rolling, and unable to urinate. His vitals, blood pressure, pulse, and respiration were all very low. I thought he had perhaps taken too much of his pain medication, but he couldn't remember. I immediately called the ambulance, informed them of my suspicions, and gave them a list of his current meds along with his last vitals. JG spent two days in the hospital after having taken too much morphine, which not only made him lethargic, but had also paralyzed his bladder so that he couldn't urinate.

JG returned home and proclaimed that I had saved his life and that he had missed me. I continued to perform the dressing changes, and eventually his legs healed. I remember how sweet he was and how attentive and lovely his family was as well.

Two maiden sisters, K and M, lived in their family home. K was skinny and constipated, while M was chubby and had diarrhea. Together they were a riot. I visited them monthly for B12 injections and pedicures.

These ladies in their mid- to late-seventies never left the house. They had a girl who cleaned and shopped for them, so they really had no need to leave. I visited them for many years and only ever saw them dressed in dusters—you know, those cotton housecoats that snap up the front. I used to tell them, "If you dress like a patient, you'll feel like a patient, and never get moving." It didn't matter if it was ninety degrees or forty below, they wore those housecoats with Daniel Green slippers. One cold winter day when I arrived, I asked them if they ever got cold in those flimsy robes, and wouldn't they like to get dressed? The answer was "No." However, they must have thought about what I said. To my surprise, on my monthly visit after Christmas, the ladies both had on brightly colored velour tracksuits. They looked so cute! I loved it!

The sisters came from a family of seven siblings. They told me that many years before, their younger sister had died of diphtheria. Their mother had to block off the front room where she died, put a black wreath on the front door, and send the body out the front window so as not to spread the disease through the house. Today's immunizations have mostly eliminated some of the horrible diseases like diphtheria, tetanus, and pertussis (whooping cough). Unfortunately, because some people are not immunizing their children, some of those once-eliminated illnesses like pertussis and measles are appearing again.

On one of my visits, I arrived to find K and M very upset. They had been hearing a chirping sound for nearly a month and were distraught at the idea that a bird was trapped in their attic, slowly dying. They said, "This poor bird just will not die, and we can't get up to the attic to see. Will you check it out?" As much as I dislike birds, I set off to see this bird trapped in the attic. As I climbed the staircase, I distinctly heard the chirp coming at regular intervals. I spotted the culprit. To my relief and theirs, the bird in question was a smoke alarm with a dead battery. I changed the battery and silenced "the bird." I was their hero that day for sure. We laughed about the incident for years to come.

I administered monthly B12 shots to E, an amazing lady in her late nineties who lived alone in an upstairs apartment. For socialization, she would go to the grocery store and visit with everyone in the store. I used to see her there quite often and would get a chance to chat with her.

One morning when I went for my scheduled visit, there was no response at the door, which was highly unusual. At this point, she was one hundred years old. Since I knew where the key was, I let myself in and started yelling for her. I heard whimpering in the hallway. There lay E, with her right leg rotated outward, and I knew immediately that she had broken her hip. She told me she had been lying there about three hours. I felt just terrible, thinking of her just lying there. I made her as comfortable as possible and called the ambulance. When I leaned over to talk to her, she said to me, "I've really done it this time, haven't I?" She knew this was it—she wasn't going to come back home—and she was right. She lived approximately two more years in an assisted-living situation. I missed her when she left and always pictured her in the doorway whenever I passed her old apartment.

Occasionally, couples make as much of an impression on me as individuals. In my travels, I frequently encountered couples who had been married forever—fifty or more years. From my experience, I have to say, it's true that couples really become one person after living together for so many years. Two couples really made a lasting impression on me: C and K, and H and IR.

C and K both had health issues. K had respiratory problems and frequently became short of breath, and C had diabetes and was losing her vision. But together they were able to cope. Where one spouse had difficulty, the other filled in. K would fill insulin syringes and read recipes to the visually challenged C so that she could administer her own injections and cook. She would help him bathe and dress, as using his arms caused him to become extremely short of breath.

These two lovely people liked to talk. We had many great conversations, especially about our hometown. K was a retired chief of police and would tell me stories about what was happening "back in the day." I was fascinated and loved hearing them.

One day, I had just finished listening to K's lungs, when all of a sudden he needed to go to the bathroom. I quickly moved, retrieved his walker, and placed it in front of him. However, I neglected to pull up the suspenders I had removed when I listened to his chest. He got halfway across the room when his pants fell to the floor around his ankles. He and his wife and I started laughing while I was quickly pulling up his pants so he could get to the bathroom in time.

K was a real joker, and he loved his wife dearly. He used to make passes at me, just kidding around. On one of my scheduled visits, I arrived and K wasn't in his usual chair. I asked C where he was, and she responded that he stayed in bed that morning. That was highly unusual for him. C and I went into the bedroom, and there was K having an extremely hard time breathing. I took his blood pressure and temperature, but in order to listen to his lungs, I had to get up on the bed. Even when he was feeling bad, he had a joke. K turned his head and said to me, "Gee, I finally got you in bed with me and I'm too sick to notice!" I called the ambulance. It turned out K had pneumonia.

Another story they shared has stuck with me all these years. When the two downsized, they bought a sweet trailer that had a Jacuzzi tub in the bathroom. One day they tried it out, and once they got in, they couldn't get out. In desperation, they finally called the fire department from the phone they'd taken with them into the bathroom. To make matters worse, one of the volunteer firemen who responded to the call was their son-in-law. The family all had a good sense of humor. C and K got a big chuckle out of the situation and loved telling me all about it.

The other memorable couple was H and IR. H had been a baker for years and had Baker's asthma, along with poor eyesight and deafness. IR was a sweetheart who had minimal arthritis, but really did very well in her old age. I met these two when H came home from the hospital after a short stay for exacerbation of COPD. At first, they were difficult to visit because he was so hard of hearing, he never heard the doorbell, and she was so afraid of intruders that she kept the door locked at all times. Finally, we arranged for me to put the dates and times of my visits on their calendar so they knew when I was coming. I visited twice a week, then once a week until he was well. When it came time to discharge him from our services, he asked me if I wanted to move into the apartment upstairs. I was in my twenties and still single at the time. I was hesitant because, one, he had been a patient and, two, I wasn't sure I could afford it. I looked at the apartment, fell in love with it, talked it over with my family, and moved.

For many years, we were upstairs-downstairs neighbors and we got along famously. Over the years, though, they both had increasing health issues. Dear IR passed away, and H went to live in assisted living near his children. After they left, my husband and I bought the double home from their children, and it's where we still live today. There are times when I go down the back stairs and think of H and IR. Recently, we were visited by their ninety-year-old daughter and were happy to show her the changes we had made to the home and reminisce about her parents.

Today, most of these extra interactions would be against the rules. I feel that this has taken a bit of the "heart" out of patient care. Beyond what I did for my patients, they have also done so much for me and remain forever in my heart.

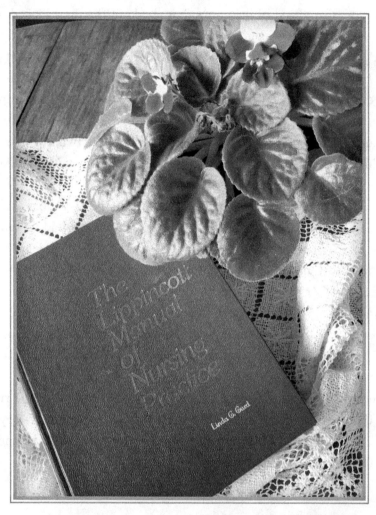

MY PERSONALIZED TEXTBOOK THAT WAS GIFTED TO ME
BY A WONDERFUL FRIEND.

TWELVE

LESSONS LEARNED:
FINAL THOUGHTS ON MY CAREER

I AM IN awe of the resilience of the human body. It's a perfect machine, so good at compensating when illness strikes. At the same time, it's a mystery. When this machine breaks down, it is time for medical professionals to become detectives, putting the puzzle pieces together in order to come up with a diagnosis and provide a course of treatment to get the body back into working order. Like any other machine, the body has a finite life expectancy. Unlike machines, though, the human body has an emotional component. Health care providers need to take the patients' feelings into account. They need to recognize the patients' "time of life" and react with the right amount of tact, compassion, and patience to provide the best level of care.

Being a nurse was pretty much a foregone conclusion for me. I was good at science, liked problem-solving, and enjoy helping others. But being a public health nurse gave me so much more than just employment at something I could do well. I learned life lessons on the job, lessons that helped me improve as a nurse, and lessons that could be applied outside the job, as well. When traveling, I am prepared. When interacting with others in a new environment, I adapt to my surroundings. When dealing with fragile individuals, I hold out a helping hand or lend a comforting shoulder. If there is a problem, I work to solve it. If something is difficult, I do the best I can in the situation. While all these lessons can be applied to the job, they can be applied to daily life too. Because the most important lesson of all is that people are people. Though they may be different from you, behave in a manner you never would, live a life that is completely foreign to you, somewhere within them is a spark of humanity that is just like yours. They get sick or injured, fear for themselves and their loved ones, and need help and understanding. For me, the best part of my job as a public health nurse was getting to know the folks I cared for. No matter how different their circumstances, they all touched me somehow, especially in their courage as they battled illness and faced death.

MY LAST DAY:
September 2013

WHEN YOU LOVE what you do, it's difficult to say goodbye. After thirty-six years of a fulfilling and satisfying career, it's my last day as a seasoned public health nurse, and it's time to turn the job over to the next generation of eager nurses. I've spent a week saying farewell to my patients—some of whom I've had for twenty or more years—had a final exit meeting with my supervisor to resolve any lingering issues, and turned in my nursing bag.

In my car are all of the extra supplies I carried "just in case." Realizing that the new nurses can use my stash, I remove the extra IV tubing, caps, extension sets, irrigation sets, suture removal sets, catheters, insertion trays, four-by-fours, Kling, and everything else a nurse might need, and turn those in as well.

After clearing my desk, I head out to my car. I get in the driver's seat and note how empty the car is without my gear. I pull out of the parking lot for the last time and start home, wondering if the new public health nurse will get the enjoyment and satisfaction from the job that I got. I hope so. It certainly was a fun ride!

ACKNOWLEDGMENTS

I WANT TO thank my dear husband, Jim, for all his love and support of me through all these years. Thanks also to my close friends—The JUGs (Just Us Girls) and my SEW sisters (Sisters Enjoying Wine)—for encouraging me to write this book. I have been telling these stories about my nursing career for many years and they all said, "You should write a book." And I finally did.

I especially want to thank Kathy Grogan for making it happen. Without her writing and organizational skills, this book would never have come to be. I believe she was able to capture the essence of my personality while helping me tell my story.

I also want to include a special thank-you to Pamela Melville—one of my SEW sisters. Your keen legal mind, constructive criticism, and editing ability were essential for the completion of this book. I could not have finished it without you!

Love you all,
Linda Laker

About the Author

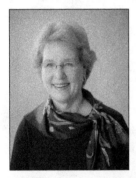

LINDA CURD LAKER lives in the small city of Hornell, New York, with her husband of twenty-nine years. She reads for pleasure with The Southern Tier Lit Chicks, whose gatherings could be mistaken for a Finger Lakes wine club. An avid quilter, Linda designs and stitches for dear friends, family, and other loved ones in an effort to capture their stories and personalities with color, material, and patterns. This is her first book.

CPSIA information can be obtained
at www.ICGtesting.com
Printed in the USA
LVHW020000220221
679523LV00002B/260